THE BEDROOM FOOL

BY

OBI ORAKWUE

THE BEDROOM FOOL

BEDROOM POLITICS SERIES

THE BEDROOM FOOL

BY OBI ORAKWUE

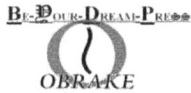

Be Your Dream Press
Imprint of Obrake USA LLC
New York, United States of America

THE BEDROOM FOOL

Library of Congress Cataloging in Publication Data
Orakwue, Obi
The Bedroom Fool/Obi Orakwue
Library of Congress Control Number 2012908996
Includes glossary of terms
ISBN 978-1-948735-00-1 (Paperback Edition)
ISBN 978-0-9856222-3-7 (E-Book Edition)
Printed in USA
First Published in USA in 2012, as E-Book
By Be Your Dream Press
Imprint of Obrake USA LLC
New York, United States of America
www.obrake.com

THE BEDROOM FOOL

Dedication

This book is dedicated to Remedies of Aging and Time, and to all who aspire to be armed with knowledge to intensify and rejuvenate their sexual health, general and bedroom wellness and harmony.

Acknowledgments

Thanks to all the people who were involved through research and or interview during the course of writing this book.

THE BEDROOM FOOL

TABLE OF CONTENTS

AUTHOR'S NOTE

In general, the politics of a relationship is a complex one. However, one aspect of the general politics of any relationship is outstanding and it is the Bedroom Politics. In this arena of politics, do not let your guard down, if you loss in this section, you lose everything. The Bedroom Fool is the real Fool of any relationship. A tight, elastic and lubricated vagina heightens the ecstasy of every inch of the travel down the vaginal canal. It is the most essential component of the magic of a come-back exploration. Vaginal tightness, weak vaginal muscles, elasticity, succulence, lubrication and general state of health and wellbeing of the vagina basically depends on the presence of and supply to the vaginal muscles of the essential nutrients, minerals, vitamins, exercise and relevant regimen. The **S**ecret to tightening, elasticizing and rejuvenating the vagina is well laid out in this guide. The general state of the vaginal wellbeing affects a person's confidence, the type of men one can keep after the first and or second sexual encounter. This is because sexual satisfaction forms more than 65% of the driving force that keeps a relationship and its intensity on and or why most couples and sex partners keep their relationship going. Enjoyable and pleasurable sexual intercourse lubricates the wheel of the complex riddle we call relationship and marriage.

Remember the old saying: "once the sex is good, most other things fall in line."

The elasticity, tightness of the vaginal walls starts to weaken and thins away as women age (genital aging) and most especially after child-birth. This may bring about low sex drive, lack of orgasm during intercourse, lack of satisfaction from sex partners and general lack of interest in sex. When the vaginal muscles are well exercised, the vaginal walls become tight thus improving the texture and feel of the vagina to the penis. You have more control of the movement of the vagina muscles during intercourse, so much so that you can clamp and clench a penis at will. You can squeeze, massage, ease and release the penis quickly and at will, and in so doing control his orgasm. The early post-virgin "click" associated with penis pull-out could be attributed to the natural strong, tight and elastic teenage vaginal muscle, after discounting vaginal flatulence. You can reclaim this power and glory by simple vaginal muscle exercise, rejuvenation, regimen, food for vaginal wellbeing and general conditioning. This guide tells you how. You just have to read it.

NO Matter How Educated, Rich and Beautiful You may be: If You are a Bedroom Fool, you will find it hard to keep partners for the long sweet haul and or keep them faithful to you, sexually. Remember, sexual faithfulness for the most part is by virtue of sexual satisfaction with one's sex partner. For the most part, sexual faithfulness is a result of culturing your partner, enslaving your partner and forcing your partner into faithfulness - voluntary and or involuntary sexual servitude by your simple acts in the bedroom during sexual intercourse. You cannot sexually enslave your partner by just dishing out non-quality sex every day, every hour with a saggy, weak, inelastic vaginal walls and unhealthy vagina.

A whole lot of good thing about the magic of healthy, tight, elastic, rejuvenated and succulent vagina is that:-

You don't have to have a great body to have a tight, elastic, healthy, succulent and rejuvenated vagina.

You don't have to be beautiful to have a healthy tight and rejuvenated vagina: You need a healthy tight, elastic, rejuvenated vagina to accentuate your beauty.

You don't have to be tall to have an elastic and tight healthy vagina.

You don't need to be intelligent to have an elastic, tight and rejuvenated healthy vagina.

You don't need to be educated to have an elastic and tight vagina.

You don't have to be rich to have an elastic, tight and rejuvenated healthy vagina. All you need to have elastic, tight, rejuvenated and healthy vagina is your willingness, readiness and the information you need to make it happen. Now with this book in hand and your desire, you have all you need to glow and radiate between the legs. The health, tightness, and elasticity of the vagina is the second most powerful chapter of a relationship after first impression and other associated impressions which one show-cases to potential suitors. So, make that impression powerful. This guide tells you how.

INTRODUCTION

Knowing what is obtainable to the benefit of the vagina, vaginal muscles and pleasurable sex will enable you to reconstruct the vaginal canal. **Remember:** The Bedroom Fool is the real Fool of any relationship.

Don't be the Bedroom Fool. Sexual enslavement, sexual servitude and sexual faithfulness have much to do with the activities in the bedroom during sexual intercourse, but most importantly the state of the vagina and vaginal walls including Tightness or Sagginess thereof, Elasticity and Lubrication. As we age, women experience hormonal changes, vaginal thinning, and sagginess, loose of elasticity, dryness, and vaginal muscle atrophy – a decrease in vaginal muscle. The said changes may bring about pain during sex, itching, soreness, and irritation. Most women are so discouraged, embarrassed, frustrated, and intimidated by these changes that they most often do not discuss it not even with a doctor. And the attendant consequence is lack of interest in sex, and abandoned sexual life. In general, women spend a good percentage of their income on anti-aging and beauty products while ignoring the health and wellbeing of their vagina. Vaginal thinning, loose of elasticity, muscle atrophy and sagginess are all part of aging that shouldn't be ignored. Sex is an essential part of enjoyment of life and relationship. Almost any woman can lure a man into sexual intercourse.

This is because to have sex with a man, a woman does not need to be sexy, beautiful, tall, rich and or attractive. All she needs is to show that she is willing and available and will say yes at the slightest invitation. However, the daunting thing is to get the same man to come back for another session. Getting the man to come back for another date depends very much on how and what he feels about the first sexual encounter.

Now, the question is:

What makes a man want to have sex with you again and again that whenever he thinks and or wants sex you come to mind? What can make any man want to go out and have sex with you again and again? Why are most men attracted to young women, irrespective of weight, beauty and class? **Fact** is that young women haven't been exposed to the ravages of time, age and other experiences that are proximate causes of vaginal loosening, sagging, inelasticity and vaginal blandness or lifelessness. A tight, elastic and lubricated vagina make the travel down the vaginal canal most pleasurable. It is the most essential component of the magic of a come-back exploration. When you have a loose, saggy, inelastic vagina it affects you and sex stop feeling like it used to and not pleasurable anymore and you may not be having orgasm. It also affects your sex partner and tolls on him, and he may start to look for an escape to the bedroom boredom. Good news is that there is therapy for the situation and you can be your vagina therapist. You just need to pay as much attention to your vaginal health and wellbeing as you pay to your general health, beauty, skin, nails and the hair. **This guide tells you how**.

PART 1

WHAT CAUSES LOOSE VAGINA?

BF

CHAPTER 1

WHAT MAKES VAGINA LOOSE?

A variety of reasons brings about vaginal loosening, loss of elasticity, sagging and general vaginal lifelessness.

The causes may range from:

- ❖ Regular sexual intercourse without adequate vaginal exercise to re-enforce the vaginal muscles
- ❖ Insertion of large objects into the vagina
- ❖ Sedentary lifestyle/lack of exercise (vaginal muscle exercise)
- ❖ Pregnancy
- ❖ Childbirth
- ❖ Hormonal changes
- ❖ Menopause
- ❖ Aging
- ❖ Vaginal muscle thinning – (Vaginal atrophy)
- ❖ Vaginal Dryness

Before going into the above-mentioned topics, let's see the vaginal wall and its structure.

THE VAGINAL WALL

The vagina is an elastic and muscular canal that runs from the vulva to the cervix. This canal has its walls made up of fibrous muscles of stratified squamous epithelial cells and tissues. The elastic nature of the vaginal canal is endowed by nature to accommodate childbirth and movements during sexual intercourse. The vagina is suspended by attachments to the perineum, pelvic floor side wall and sacrum by smooth muscles (vaginal muscles) made up of collagen and elastin fibers. The vaginal wall is divided into two parts: the front (anterior) wall and the back (posterior) wall. The anterior wall is about 7cm in length and runs (7 cm) from the vulva to the posterior wall. The posterior wall is about 9cm. The total length of the vagina canal is about 16cm. The length and diameter of the vaginal canal alters/changes by stretching manifold beyond the normal length and size during childbirth and sexual intercourse. Along the vaginal wall are folds (ridges), sometimes called the vaginal rugae. The unfolding of the rugae aids the elastic nature of the vaginal canal by creating more surface area. The layers of muscle in the stratified squamous epithelium of the vaginal wall include:

Mucosa – non-keratinized stratified squamous epithelium

Sub-mucosa – under the mucosa

Muscularis – smooth muscles (intermixed with sub-mucosa and adventitia)

The adventitia is made up of mainly elastin fibers which are responsible for the elastic nature of the vaginal canal. Elastin is a structural protein responsible for the elasticity of most body tissues.

REGULAR SEXUAL INTERCOURSE

In other to accuse regular sexual intercourse as a culprit in vaginal muscle loosening and loose vagina, let's have a look at what happens during sexual intercourse. During sexual arousal the vagina expands in both length and width. The elasticity allows the vaginal canal to stretch during sexual intercourse and during birth of offspring. During sexual arousal and eventual intercourse, the vaginal elastic folds (ridges) called rugae unfolds to provide more surface area to support the extension and stretching of the vaginal wall. In the arousal and the actual intercourse, the vagina lengthens to about 10cm on the average, though it can continue to lengthen and expand in width to accommodate the pressure and size of the invading penis and or object. As the vaginal wall lengthens, the diameter of the opening alters, clamping the invading penis or object to provide tightness. This is true in the case of a tight and healthy vagina. The rugae are transverse epithelial cells and tissues. The elasticity and strength of the rugae and vaginal muscle layers including the mucosa, sub-mucosa, muscularis and adventitia, though are sustainable but are spendable.

This means that the more they are put in use without adequate replenishment and or re-enforcement through adequate care and exercise, the weaker and less elastic they tend to become.

This type of vaginal wall and vaginal muscle loosening affects mainly young women in active sex phase and of child bearing age. The saying; "she is young but has a vagina of an 'old' woman" is true to this end. The interpretation of this verse is not entirely consistent with: "regular sexual intercourse is not healthy and or loosens your vaginal wall muscles".

However, the interpretation may be consistent with: "regular sexual intercourse without adequate care and regular vaginal muscle exercise is not healthy, as it may loosen your vaginal wall muscles." When the vaginal wall muscles are weak, the pelvic floor muscle is also weak. The PC muscle (pubococcygeal muscle) is the muscle that contracts when a woman has orgasm. When this muscle is weak and unable to contract, orgasm cannot be attained. Therefore, majority of women who have regular sexual intercourse cannot boost of quality sex and or regular orgasm. Example are women in the sex trade, most of them interviewed during the course of writing this book confessed to have not had orgasm in years despite having 5 to 10 sex sessions every day. When you exercise the wall muscles of the vaginal canal and the PC muscle (pubococcygeal muscle), you will enjoy quality sex and have powerful orgasm. This is even clearer as clinical research and statistics have shown a powerful direct correlation between weak vaginal wall muscles, flaccid PC muscle (pubococcygeal muscle), lack of orgasm, and lack of vaginal muscle exercise. The PC muscle (pubococcygeal muscle) sometimes called the love muscle forms part of the woman's pelvic floor. The pelvic floor is a group of muscles that are present in the pelvic cavity, supporting the bladder, uterus, vaginal canal and other organs in the pelvic cavity. PC muscle (pubococcygeal muscle) exercise, vaginal wall muscle exercise tightens the vagina, by tightening and toning the PC muscle (pubococcygeal muscle) and the vaginal wall muscles, giving you a lot of power and control between your legs.

So? Enjoy your sex as regularly as you can, but, engage in an equally regular vaginal muscle exercise to re-enforce your PC (love) muscles and be ready for an equally next quality sex session. Sex is good after all.

INSERTION OF LARGE OBJECTS INTO THE VAGINA

Large objects such as toys used during masturbation can weaken the muscle of the vaginal wall, as they undergo regular lengthening and widening. This is relatively true even with effective regular PC and vaginal muscle exercise. When large toys and objects are used regularly during masturbation, the vaginal wall and opening somewhat get trained and used to a particular lengthening and widening, so much so that any smaller invading object and or penis may feel 'lost' and without friction (tightness) in the canal.

However, any invading object and or penis that is of the same or larger size of the regular (perpetrator) large object will without doubt fit the tightness of the canal, if effective regular PC and vaginal muscle exercise is in place.

SEDENTARY LIFE/LACK OF EXERCISE

Just as in most other general body health, sedentary life is not good for the health of the vaginal wall muscles and the PC muscle (pubococcygeal muscle). If the vaginal muscles are not regularly exercised, it gets flabby and thus loose vagina.

PREGNANCY

During pregnancy, a lot of hormonal changes take place in a woman's body including increase in the body progesterone, estrogen and prolactin. The pelvic floor muscle also weakens during pregnancy. The pelvic floor muscle supports the uterus, urethra, rectum, bladder and the vaginal canal. The weakening of the pelvic floor muscle may lead to vaginal prolapse. Vaginal prolapse is when one of the pelvic organs falls into the vaginal canal. Organs that may fall into the vaginal canal if the pelvic floor muscle is weak include the rectum and the bladder. The bladder falls into the vaginal canal if the front vaginal wall muscle is weaker, and the rectum falls into the vaginal canal if the back vaginal wall muscle is weaker. Changes during pregnancy also include enlargement of the reproductive organs, reproductive bodies, general body enlargement and other associated stretches. The enlargements are in preparation for the development of the fetus and eventual delivery. One of the most used proteins of the body system for the body enlargement and stretches is the elastin (a structural protein) and collagen. Elastin is most abundant in the skin and vaginal walls. Elastin is responsible for the elastic nature of the vaginal canal and vaginal wall. It is also true that during pregnancy, physical activity and exercise are greatly reduced. Pregnant women are susceptible to urinary incontinence. Incontinence is the loss of bladder muscle control, and urinary incontinence is the inability to stop urine leakage from the bladder. If the pelvic muscle floor is weak, the PC muscle (pubococcygeal muscle) is weak, the vaginal wall elastin is depleted, the Vagina will become loose without resistance.

CHILD DELIVERY/BIRTH

Child birth is one of the most common causes of Loose Vagina. It is the biggest culprit of loose vagina in women of child bearing age. During natural vaginal birth, the vagina stretches to accommodate the head and body of the baby. The extent of the stretch depends on the size of the baby. The stretching is as a result of the pelvic muscles and the vaginal muscles. With successive births, the vagina loosens. However, the pelvic muscles and the vaginal wall muscles like most other muscles in the human body are resilient and elastic. This means they have the ability to return to normalcy after stretches, relaxations and contractions. The return to normalcy of a loose vagina from child birth requires a combination of vaginal muscle exercise, care and therapy.

MENOPAUSE

Menopause comes with associated hormonal changes including decrease in estrogen levels, vaginal dryness, loss of elasticity in the vaginal walls, and the ultimately loose vagina. Decrease in estrogens levels in a woman's hormonal system causes the vaginal walls to thin away and become inflamed, and the vaginal walls loose strength and elasticity. It also depletes vaginal natural lubrication.

The natural lubrication of the vagina comes from the Bartholin's gland, located near the vaginal opening. The epithelial cells and tissues of a healthy vaginal wall also supplies moisture to the vaginal canal. Vaginal dryness, a symptom of menopause is well associated with unhealthy vaginal wall. The vaginal wall is made up of stratified squamous epithelial fibrous muscles. Menopause therefore causes vaginal muscle atrophy and loose vagina.

AGING

Aging of all sorts brings about associated decrease and loss of health including loss of vaginal elasticity, strength and weakening of pelvic floor muscles. As we age, blood flow and blood circulation decrease and muscle mass and tone also decrease including vaginal wall muscles and the pelvic floor muscle. Older women also have less lubricated vagina, this causes dryness and itching.

When the vagina is dry, inelastic, and weak, it inevitably becomes loose.

VAGINAL ATROPHY OR ATROPHIC VAGINITIS

Vaginal atrophy normally occurs in post-menopausal stage of most women's life and also in women of all ages with extremely sedentary lifestyle. Vaginal atrophy is mostly associated with thinning of vaginal walls. One of the proximate causes of vaginal atrophy is drop in estrogen production. Estrogen treatments and replacement may decrease vaginal atrophic symptoms. The elderly and inactive/sedentary people are most susceptible to vaginal atrophy.

As we age, blood flow and blood circulation decrease and muscle mass and tone also decreases including vagina wall muscles and the pelvic floor muscle. Testosterone, progesterone and estrogen are the chief sex hormones which fall out of normal balance as we age. When one of the hormones is out of balance, it affects the balance of the rest of other hormones. Testosterone is more closely associated with a person's muscle mass. When the estrogen levels of the body decreases, it invariably decreases the normal level of testosterone level and thins away the muscle.

Atrophic vaginitis may also affect young women of child-bearing age due to breastfeeding, hysterectomy or chemo-radiation therapies for cancer. The structural changes to the vaginal walls is often associated with symptoms such as itching, burning, swelling and vaginal dryness, severe pain and discomfort during sex.

Though atrophic vaginitis commonly causes discomfort and pain, however, overall, it is an otherwise benign vaginal health condition. Atrophic vaginitis may be a prelude to bacterial infections including candida, or yeast infections, and urinary tract infections.

ASSOCIATED CONSEQUENCES OF LOOSE VAGINA

INCONTINENCE

Incontinence is the loss of bladder muscle control. That is when one can no longer control the muscles of the bladder. And urinary incontinence is the inability to stop urine leakage from the bladder. Incontinence can deny one of sleep and leave you exhausted. Incontinence keeps sufferers from travelling or makes travel awkward and keep victims from enjoying physical activity. Some victims are discouraged from leaving their homes and most often do not discuss it with anyone and never seek help. Incontinence occurs when any part of the urinary system fails to function.

TYPES OF INCONTINENCE

Overactive bladder

Stress incontinence

Overflow incontinence

Mixed incontinence

Women are more susceptible to incontinence because the structure of their internal organs is different to make provision for childbirth.

Causes of incontinence include Pregnancy, childbirth, and decreased levels of estrogen which are proximate or collateral causes of weakened pelvic floor muscles. Weak pelvic floor muscles make organs such as the bladder, urethra, and uterus to stay out of place or prolapse.

Characteristics of Different Incontinence(s)

URGE INCONTINENCE or OVERACTIVE BLADDER

- ✓ Wet themselves as soon as they have an urge
- ✓ Frequent and or wakeful nights to urinate
- ✓ Use the bathroom every two hours in the least
- ✓ Feel they have a weak bladder.
- ✓ Each drink of coffee, cola, or alcohol seems to cause urination out of proportion to the amount they actually consumed
- ✓ Wet their bed at night
- ✓ Leak urine during sexual intercourse

STRESS INCONTINENCE

- ✓ Leak urine when they cough, sneeze, laugh or anything that can shake the body
- ✓ Frequent bathroom visit, in an effort to avert urinary accidents
- ✓ Avoid physical exercise as it may cause leaks
- ✓ Wet their beds at nights and restful hours/sessions
- ✓ Sometimes leak urine when they get up from a chair without
- ✓ knowing they leaked

OVERFLOW INCONTINENCE

- ✓ Frequent and dribble night and day urination
- ✓ Take a long time to urinate and have a weak dribbling (inconsistent/irregular) stream
- ✓ Urinate small amounts of urine and never feel completely empty afterward
- ✓ Feel the urge to urinate, but sometimes can't

MIXED INCONTINENCE

Combination of all the above signs and symptoms

RECTAL INCONTINENCE

Rectal incontinence is as a result of loose rectal wall muscles and anal muscles. Loose vaginal wall muscle may sometimes be associated with loose rectal wall muscles. In rectal incontinence, feces or stool pass down the rectum and out the anus without control.

VAGINAL PROLAPSE

The pelvic floor muscle supports the uterus, urethra, rectum, bladder and the vaginal canal. Weakening of the pelvic floor muscle may lead to vaginal prolapse. Vaginal prolapse is when one of the pelvic organs falls into the vaginal canal. Organs that may fall into the vaginal canal if the pelvic floor muscle is weak include the uterus, rectum and the bladder. The bladder falls into the vaginal canal if the front vaginal wall muscle is weaker, and the rectum falls into the vaginal canal if the back vaginal wall muscle is weaker. Weak vaginal muscles, weak pc muscles, insufficient muscle tone, age, pregnancy, family history, and hormonal status all contribute to the development of pelvic organ prolapse or vaginal prolapse.

VAGINAL FLATULENCE OR FLATUS VAGINALIS

The expulsion of trapped air from the vagina is called vaginal flatulence. The air may enter the vaginal canal during penetration, oral stimulation or during regular exercise. This may occur during sexual intercourse or after sexual intercourse as the penis pulls out or after the penis has pulled out. The air is usually odorless and is not waste gases such as methane. This however, is not a medical concern and or any cause for alarm, though, it may be embarrassing. In some rear cases, vaginal flatulence may mean a medical condition that may require attention.

DEAD SEX DRIVE

TOTAL LACK OF INTEREST IN SEX

Women with loose vagina oftentimes do not have interest in having sex, having lost all and any sex drive they have otherwise had.

PROBABLE CAUSES OF DEAD SEX DRIVE

The lack of interest in having sexual intercourse may be from any of the following reasons:

Lack of Orgasm Over Time

The end point of sexual intercourse is being able to reach orgasm. Orgasm is the gratification of sexual intercourse. The climax of sexual intercourse is reaching and maintaining orgasm, that point when every cell, tissue and organ of the body make up is in ecstasy. When a woman has loose vagina – weak vaginal wall muscles, weak PC muscle (pubococcygeal muscle), it is impossible to attain orgasm. The PC muscle (pubococcygeal muscle) sometimes called the love muscle is the muscle that contracts to give orgasm. When the PC muscle (pubococcygeal muscle) is relaxed, flabby and therefore unable to contract, orgasm is impossible. And when the PC muscle is very weak

and flabby, it contracts with very minimal force and give very weak and non-pleasurable orgasm. This is true even when you employ the services of a professional gigolo who knows how best to take a woman to heaven, to paradise. Well, because he is a professional, he may be able to take you to heaven, but, you will not enter the paradise. In this case, that is when the PC muscle reluctantly contracts. See how serious it is? Do not despair, hope is within reach, right in hands, in the next few pages you will be reading the solution to your loose vagina. Stay tuned!

Unsatisfactory Sex Sessions

With a loose vagina, you may be unable to satisfy your sex partner(s), irrespective of your beauty and sophistication. A tight vagina makes every inch of the travel down the vaginal canal most pleasurable. A tight vagina and strong vaginal walls also makes a woman feel every inch of the thrust a sex partner makes as he travels and wriggles within. The feel of a tight vagina with strong vaginal wall muscles is mesmerizing to all participants. With a tight vagina and horned vaginal wall muscle and PC muscle (pubococcygeal muscle), you will have control of your sexual intercourse sessions. You will be able to clamp and clench the penis at will. You can clamp, squeeze, massage, ease and release the penis quickly or slowly and at will, and in so doing control his and your orgasm.

Single Session Interest

When the vagina is loose, the best one can get from most partners is a one-night stand or on session stand. A tight, elastic and lubricated vagina makes every inch of the travel down the vaginal canal pleasurable. It is the most essential component of the magic of a come-back and pleasurable exploration.

When one has a loose, saggy, inelastic vagina it affects you and sex stop feeling like it used to and not pleasurable anymore and you may not be having orgasm. It also affects your sex partner and tolls on him, and he may start to look for an escape to the boredom. Good news is that there is therapy for the situation and you can be your vagina therapist.

Avoidance After a Sex Session

Ejaculation during sex sessions does not mean enjoying the sex and or orgasm. Orgasm in essence has stages and quality. The ejaculation during intercourse with a loose vagina is totally different with one of tight, lubricated, rejuvenated vagina.

Loose vagina may cost you your sex partners. Tighten up now. Help is in your hand.

Vaginal Dryness

Dryness is a symptom of an unhealthy vagina and could be caused by a variety of reasons. The reasons may range from decrease in hormonal balance/level, to use of certain products during vaginal cleaning sessions and or other sessions.

Decrease in estrogens levels in a woman's hormonal system causes the vaginal walls to thin away and become inflamed, and the vaginal walls loss strength and elasticity. It also depletes vaginal natural lubrication. The natural lubrication of the vagina comes from the Bartholin's gland, located near the vaginal opening. The epithelial cells and tissues of a healthy vaginal wall also supplies moisture to the vaginal canal.

Dry vagina is associated with weak vaginal wall muscle and PC muscle (pubococcygeal muscle) and therefore loose vagina. A dry vagina is rarely an enjoyable vagina during intercourse. The wetter the vagina, the better the sex.

Dry vagina may bring about itching and severe pain during sexual intercourse and this may dissuade a woman from having sex and eventually to total lack of interest in sexual intercourse. The next few pages give solution to this problem. Stay tuned.

Severe Pain During Sexual Intercourse

Due to dryness and other associated problems a woman may experience severe pain and itching in her vagina and the pain intensifies during sexual intercourse and this discourages lots of victims from having sex. In other cases, severe vaginal pain may be due to a condition some experts called Vaginismus, which is a form of vaginal disorder whereby the muscles around the opening of the vagina contracts involuntarily and closes off the vaginal opening. When this happens, any form of vaginal penetration such as by the penis, object, even finger(s) becomes very painful

Vaginal Prolapse

Vaginal prolapse is the climax of a loose vaginal wall muscle and weak pelvic floor muscle. At this stage one or more of the pelvic organs may fall into the vaginal canal. It may be uterus, rectum and the bladder. At this stage the vagina is entirely loose. Most women at this stage of vaginal disaster have given up having sex.

Incontinence

The lack of control over the urinary bladder is embarrassing in the least. Women with urinary incontinence sometimes leak urine during sexual intercourse and this is extremely embarrassing. This may cause lots of women to abstain from sex without seeking help. Help is in your hands. Stay tuned for the next few pages and chapters.

Vaginal Flatulence

This is not any problem and or medical condition in itself. It is simply the expulsion of air from the vaginal canal. However, this expulsion of air is accompanied with some noise which may occur once or several times during sexual intercourse or after the sexual intercourse. In cases where it happens several times during or after intercourse, some women may find it very embarrassing, and this may sometimes

dissuade some from having sex.

PART 2

HOW TO DETERMINE A LOOSE VAGINA

BF

CHAPTER 2

WHAT CONSTITUTES A LOOSE VAGINA?
HOW TO DETERMINE A LOOSE VAGINA

In the previous chapter, we discussed causes of loose vagina without pointing out what actually constitute a loose vagina. What are the pertinent signs of a loose vagina? From the male sex partner point of view this question and the answer may remain relative in that what constitutes a loose vagina to a small, medium, and or large sized man differs. This is so, noting that: to a male sex partner the tightness of a vagina is the mere degree of friction (discounting friction due to dryness). However, this may not stand at all times, in that a vagina may be tight due to the size of the invading penis, but the feel of the vaginal texture may indicate a loose or lack of vaginal wall strength. The main determinants of a loose and or tight vagina therefore could only be deciphered through some physical examinations, and answers to questionnaires provided by the patient. In determining whether a vagina is loose or tight, we must remember that all involved in making a vagina loose and or tight are the muscles in play including the PC muscle (pubococcygeal muscle) and the vaginal wall muscles.

The following are factors you may employ to determine whether your vagina is loose and or tight:

PHYSICAL EXAMINATION

Does the Vagina Close Completely When You are Relaxed and Un-aroused?

The vaginal opening is elastic and should be reasonably closed when you are un-aroused. Remember what happens during arousal before the actual penetration and intercourse.

During arousal of all sorts, the vaginal wall lengthens, and becomes lubricated, and as the walls lengthens the vaginal opening opens and wets in anticipation for the visitor. Accordingly, in the absence of arousal, the opening of the vagina should be completely closed. Now the degree of closure and or openness determines the degree of tightness and or loose state of the vagina.

Can You Insert 3 or More of Your Fingers in Your Vagina with Little or no Resistance?

If you are able to insert one or two of your fingers into your vagina and feel the tightness, you are good. However, if you can fit in more than 3 of your fingers into your vagina, then you may have a loose vagina.

Can You Hold and Squeeze, Clamp and Clench the Penis as it moves inside the Vagina?

Yes? Good! However, the inability to do this act may not in itself be a sign of loose vagina in that the lack may be as a result of lack of exercise and expertise. But, if you have a strong vaginal wall muscles, you should be able to hold or clamp the penis without being able to clench, squeeze and or massage it.

The tightness and or looseness of a Vagina wholly depend on the vaginal wall muscles and the pelvic floor muscles.

Kegel Balls

Insert a Kegel ball, or cone into the vagina and see if you can hold it and for how long. If you are able to hold for a reasonable length of time standing, then you may not be loose. It you are able to move the ball back and forth the vaginal canal sitting down, that may equally be a sign of *'not loose'*. For the sake of this test, holding the cone for 5 – 20 seconds while standing is not bad. And being able to move the ball back and forth the vaginal canal for 5- 20 seconds is equally not a bad start. Do them for 2 to 5 sessions. The size and weight of the Kegel ball to be used for this test depends on your size, and whether or not you have used Kegel balls before. Try and see if you are able to hold the cone and or the ball standing with your legs closed together, with your legs open and with your legs wide open. We will discuss this exercise in more detail in the next chapters.

Vaginal Manometer OR Vaginal Perineometer

Pelvic floor muscle tone and vaginal muscle strength may be estimated using a device called perineometer or vaginal manometer. Perineometer (vaginal manometer) measures the vaginal air pressure generated by voluntary contraction(s) of the pelvic floor muscles/vaginal muscle. When inserted, the patient squeezes the pelvic muscles as explained in the pages of this book. The result will suggest how much she needs to train and how much she will benefit from strengthening the vaginal muscles using the Kegel exercises.

The perineometer was developed by Dr. Arnold Kegel. Another device for checking the love muscle tone is the electromyograph (EMG) perineometers. The device works by measuring the electrical activity in the pelvic floor muscles and may be more effective in this purpose. Gynecological examination by a professional may also help to establish the state of the PC muscles.

OTHER DETERMINANTS OF LOOSE VAGINA

Lack of Orgasm

If you are unable to attain orgasm during arousal, masturbation and or sexual intercourse, you definitely have loose vagina. It is good to note that the looseness and tightness of a vagina is dependent on the functionality of the vaginal wall muscles and the PC muscle (love muscle). <u>In other to have orgasm under any circumstance, the PC muscle needs to **contract**, and that is what makes orgasm possible</u>. When the PC muscle is relaxed, flabby and unable to contract, then orgasm is impossible. The PC muscle is a member of the pelvic floor muscles. When the PC muscle is flabby and weak, most other muscles are weak and flabby to the same and or varying degree. Lack of orgasm therefore is a sign of loose vagina.

Takes Longer than Normal To Achieve Orgasm

In this case orgasm is attainable but delays unusually. This means that the PC Muscle and vaginal wall muscles are not functioning properly and needs to be horned, exercised and trained to optimize functionality.

You Need Larger Object and or Penis To Achieve Orgasm?

If you now need larger sex toy(s) for your masturbation sessions and or larger penis than usual to be able to reach and maintain orgasm, then your love muscle is weak and needs to be exercised and toned. Your vagina is loose, or at least less tight than it usually should.

Incontinence: Do you leak urine when you cough, sneeze, laugh, yawn and jump, walk fast, run, etc.? If so, then your pelvic floor muscles are weak and it is a factor in loose vagina.

Vaginal Dryness: A Loose vagina is an unhealthy vagina. The vaginal wall oozes moisture into the vaginal canal during arousal and sexual intercourse. The lack of lubrication is interpretable as an unhealthy state of the vaginal wall muscles. Half of vaginal lubrication is provided by moisture from the vaginal wall muscles. It is also true that vaginal dryness could be caused by other culprits such as decreased estrogen production, etc. **In all**, the tightness and or flabbiness of your vagina depend on the health of your pelvic floor muscles, PC muscle and vaginal wall muscles. Loose vagina can befall women of all ages – young and old.

****

PART 3

MEASURES AND CORRECTION FOR LOOSE VAGINA

VAGINAL TIGHTENING

BF

CHAPTER 3

VAGINAL TIGHTENING

Now it has been determined that you have a loose vagina and or that you need to tighten and strengthen your vaginal wall muscle and your love muscle. We will discuss remedial measures to tighten and strengthen the pelvic floor muscles, PC muscle, and vaginal wall muscle, improve orgasm and empower your sex life. Ways by which the PC muscle, vaginal wall muscles, and the vagina could be tightened includes:

- ❖ Vaginal Muscle Exercise
- ❖ Vaginal Tightening Creams and Sprays
- ❖ Vaginal Rejuvenation Procedure
- ❖ Hormone Replacement
- ❖ Food for Vaginal Tightening and General Wellbeing
- ❖ Herbal Remedies

VAGINAL MUSCLE EXERCISE

Vaginal muscle exercise(s) is the easiest and least expensive way to tone, and condition the vaginal wall muscle, and tighten the vaginal opening and vaginal canal. To reap the benefits of these exercises you need to be patient and religiously follow the steps involved in the stages of the exercise.

In tightening your vaginal wall muscle and PC muscle you will improve your orgasm, making orgasm as strong, intense and satisfying as you never thought possible, have quality sex and generally enhance, empower and re-ignite your sex life and that of your sex partner. Vaginal muscle exercise could be done at anytime and anywhere and it is not strenuous. Some women prefer the medical and or surgical procedures that cost thousands of dollars for reasons that may range from immediate result to being ill informed. **Good thing** about vaginal muscle exercises is that they do not cause any harm to the body and they are very affordable and within the reach of every woman who desires to have a tight vagina, improved sex life and enhanced and intense orgasm. The impediment to the fruitful result of these vaginal exercises is that most women would not have the will power and endurance to continue doing them until they get results. If done regularly and correctly they often work, and work abundantly.

KEGEL EXERCISE

Kegel Exercise is attributed to Dr. Arnold Kegel who discovered the simple exercise. In the 1940's Dr. Kegel found out that one can actually tighten the vagina and strengthen the vaginal muscles by exercising the PC muscle and pelvic floor muscles. The simple squeeze-and-hold vaginal exercises specifically designed to target pelvic floor strengthening then become known as *Kegels*. Kegel exercises have long been accepted as one of the best method to tighten your PC muscle and vagina.

Kegels is good for women of all ages. It is often advisable when one starts at a young age to do Kegels.

The first thing to be done when starting Kegels is to identify the right muscle to be exercised and toned. This is good because it is very easy to bring other, irrelevant muscles into play while doing Kegels. To isolate the pelvic muscle and target the right muscle, you must:

- ✓ not pull in your tummy
- ✓ not squeeze your legs together
- ✓ not tighten your buttocks
- ✓ not hold your breath

Remember the sensation you feel when you have to use the washroom/bathroom to urinate, and how you suck it in and hold it. The very muscle you use to hold back the urine is the relevant muscle. This is a Kegel. **Now pretend** that you have to use the washroom desperately, now contract your relevant muscles to hold it. Did you do it right? If so, that is Kegels and you can do Kegels whenever you want and wherever you are. They are one of the best exercises you need to do if you want to make your vaginal muscles stronger and your vagina tighter.

Now let's do the real one. Do you have the urge to urinate? Yes? Good. Go to the washroom and let the tap (urine) on.

Now stop the flow of urine. Hold it! Now let go, let urine flow again.

Hold it again. Hold!

Now let flow again.

The muscle you use to hold the urine flow is the PC muscle you need to exercise and tone. Provided you did not pull your stomach muscles, squeeze your legs together, tighten your buttocks and or hold your breath.

Remember, don't do this often, it is not safe as an exercise during urinary urge.

To Further Identify the PC Muscle, Do the following:

Sit on a clean toilet and spread your legs as wide as you can, then urinate and empty your bladder completely. Insert a finger into the vagina and contract the same muscle as if you want to stop the flow of urine, feel the contractions.

Step 1

Squeeze and hold the PC muscle for 4 seconds. Relax and repeat the process.

Step 2

Contract and release the PC muscle about 10 to 12 times.

Step 3

Contract the PC muscle and hold for 10 to 15 seconds. This is somewhat how Kegels work. However, for comprehensive details, you should read more literature on Kegel exercises.

You need to do this as many times as possible every day. On the average do 20 sessions of 10 contraction, totaling 200 or 300 as the case may be. **Remember,** the result is never immediate; you need to be patient and persistent. Sometimes it takes at least a couple of weeks if not months for the result to manifest. And you will be able to enjoy intense orgasm, clamp, and clench and massage your partner's penis and enslave him sexually.

Motivation and determination are the very key for success with Kegels. Exercises provide resistance. Remember just like ordinary exercise, going to the gym, you do not see any tangible result in the first week or two, you need to continue going to the gym until you tone your body muscles and achieve the desired body tone and shape, the same applies to Kegels and your PC muscle. Because Kegels is an invisible exercise that can be done anywhere, whether you're alone, talking to a friend, or in a crowd of people, in a grocery store and in the subway, etc., does not make it any different from any other exercise. In an effort to perfect and or make Kegel exercises more effective, devices, objects and methods have been designed to aid in Kegels.

Some Kegel devices include:

- ➢ Kegel Balls
- ➢ Jade eggs
- ➢ Duotone Balls
- ➢ Smart Balls
- ➢ Pleasure Balls
- ➢ Vaginal Cones

The balls and cones differ in sizes and weight. They have small, medium and large sizes and weight categories. The one you use as a person depends on your size, and stage in the exercise. They can be made from metal, plastic, stone, marble, ceramic and silicone. Balls made from metal, ceramics and stone are somewhat safer as they do not absorb bacteria. The balls are sterilized before using. You can sterilize the balls using hot water or steam. Balls and cones made of plastic are often light in weight and need to be made heavier with some added weights inside the balls. Metal balls are hollow balls and may also contain ball bearings inside for added weight.

Silicone and rubber balls are soft and can be squeezed to acquire added resistance. When you insert the Kegel balls into the vagina, you need to contract the PC muscles to hold them in place. The movement of the PC muscles can also move the balls back and forth while sitting down, this in itself may provide some form of arousal or stimulation for some women.

However, a beginner may want to start off with large balls as they are easier to grasp and hold with the PC muscle. While standing, insert the ball into the vagina and squeeze/contract the PC muscle to hold it in place. Try holding the ball for say ten seconds. Then repeat the exercise ten to 30 times a day, giving a total of 200 to 300 contractions. It is very important to do the exercises daily to achieve results. After your muscles have improved, you can move on to smaller balls, which are a little more difficult to hold and needs experienced muscle to hold them.

POSITIONS TO EMPLOY WHILE EXERCISING WITH KEGEL BALLS/DEVICES

You can use the balls to exercise in different positions including:

Sitting

In this position, open your legs and insert the ball. Close your legs and start to use the same muscle you use to hold the flow of urine to try and move the ball inside you, back and forth for as many times as you could. Do sessions per day.

Standing

Insert the ball inside your vaginal canal and close your legs and try to hold the ball from falling. Hold as long as you can, relax the muscle and contract again. Do this session as many times as you can per day. Try doing it with your legs open and then wide open and see if you can hold the ball in place.

Squatting

While squatting with legs wide open, insert the ball into the vagina and use your vaginal muscles to push the ball inner into your vaginal canal. Repeat as many times as possible.

CONES

Most vaginal cones are made of stainless steel, marble and ceramics and most vaginal cones have the shape of a regular tampon. Vaginal cones also come in different sizes and weights. Cones are better employed in Kegels while standing.

OTHER METHODS

ELECTRICAL STIMULATION

This is sometimes called Neuro-electrical stimulation. A probe of this device inserted into the pelvic floor generates electric current which contracts and relaxes the vaginal muscle.

NEOCONTROL

This method employs a chair which generates a magnetic field that stimulates the pelvic floor.

OTHER EXERCISES FOR THE PELVIC FLOOR MUSCLES

What is the Pelvic Floor?

The pelvic floor is that point in the pelvic region of the body where all the connective tissues and muscles that support all the organs of the pelvis connect. And the pelvic floor muscles are the muscles that are connected to the pelvic floor. Some of the muscles include:

- ➤ Vaginal muscle
- ➤ Rectal Muscle
- ➤ Urethra
- ➤ Uterus
- ➤ Perineum muscle

PERINEAL MASSAGE

The name given to this exercise arises from the perineum, which as seen from the topical body, is the skin that connects/between the rectum and the vagina. From the inside, the perineal body stretches inwards from the perineum area and provides the insertion point/base of the other muscles (eight muscles) that forms the pelvic floor. When the perineum is massaged, blood circulation is increased, and more blood flows to the pelvic floor improving the health of the pelvic floor muscles.

To massage the perineum, you insert oiled thumbs into the base of the vaginal opening and press downwards towards the back/spine. Do this as many times a week as you can. This massage improves the flexibility or elasticity of the pelvic floor muscles. Perineal massage involves lubricating the thumbs and inserting them inside the base of the vagina, then exerting downward pressure toward the back of the spine. A person's tolerance will increase as she practices, and the pelvic floor will become more flexible. This can be done by any woman seeking to improve pelvic floor flexibility. Perineal massage is especially good for pregnant women because it combines breathing with downward pressure thereby improving flexibility, which is particularly helpful during birth.

SQUATTING EXERCISE

This exercise is easy. You can squat as many times and many sessions as you can per day. It helps to strengthen the pelvic floor and the pelvic floor muscles. Squatting is good for women of all ages.

****

BF

CHAPTER 4

ROLE OF HORMONES IN VAGINAL TIGHTENING

Hormonal changes in a woman's body may bring about vaginal dryness and loosening. Hormonal changes may occur in young and or older women. However, older people are most prone to decrease in body hormone production. The hormone in play in this respect includes estrogen and DHEA. Though DHEA itself is neither a hormone nor a vitamin, however, it is a precursor, aid and or regulator for sex hormones.

As noted in the previous chapter, decrease in estrogens levels in a woman's hormonal system causes the vaginal walls to thin away and become inflamed, and the vaginal walls loss strength and elasticity. It also depletes vaginal natural lubrication. One of the proximate causes of vaginal atrophy is a drop in estrogen production. Estrogen treatments and replacement may decrease vaginal atrophic symptoms and vaginal dryness.

DHEA or Dehydroepiandrosterone is a steroid hormone produced by the body to create both male and female hormones. DHEA is secreted naturally in the body by the adrenal glands.

DHEA and estrogen hormone levels in the body tends to peak in the twenties and decline as people get older.

DHEA is converted in the body to both the female hormone, estrogen and the male hormone testosterone. Levels of DHEA decline naturally with age and this can lead to decreased estrogen levels and subsequently atrophic vaginitis, vaginal dryness, vaginal itching, decreased sex drive, decreased libido and ultimately loose vagina. DHEA is available over the counter (OTC) in most drug stores in USA. However, it is good to remember that hormones are precision substances in that at any point, hormones require the proper balance to work effectively. And when you overdose on them, the resulting imbalance may cause health problems rather than improve them. You are therefore advised to consult an experienced professional before employing hormonal replacement therapy and make sure you have the correct dosage and are in good health. Sometimes on and off consumption of supplements may be safe. However, you can in the alternative engage in consuming natural foods, herbs, and vitamins that are rich in these hormones. Consuming foods and herbs rich in estrogen is entirely harmless. However, consumption must be persistent to achieve desired result. In the next chapter we will be discussing foods and vitamins that aid vaginal tightening.

For more information on Hormonal changes and hormonal imbalance **See the Book: BEDROOM LOGIC**

BF

CHAPTER 5

FOODS, HERBS AND VITAMIN
FOR VAGINAL TIGHTENING

MANJAKANI OR OAK GALL

The word Manjakani is Malay language for Oak Gall. Manjakani or oak gall is popularly consumed in Malaysia, Indonesia and South East Asia by women after birth and generally by nursing mothers. It is believed and proven that the tonic herbal drink has positive effect on toning and tightening vaginal muscles after childbirth. Oak Galls is produced by the activities of stinging wasps on the leaves of the oak tree. Oak Gall is a round hard ball which is formed from chemical reaction arising from secretions by various insects most especially the stinging wasp as they penetrate the leaves of Oak tree leaves to lay eggs and other activities.Oak Gall is very rich in calcium, iron, vitamins A and C, tannins, tannic acid, gallic acid, fiber, protein and carbohydrates. Oak gall has astringent properties that help in toning, tightening and firming the vaginal wall muscles. It restores vaginal wall elasticity and tone. In addition, assists in reducing vaginal discharge called leucorrhoea which causes bad vaginal odor and also eliminates vaginal itching. Its antiseptic properties are very effective in fighting vaginal yeast, bacterial and fungal infection.

CURCUMA COMOSA

Curcuma comosa is a species of flowering plant of the Ginger family. The herb is a native of Asia. It is most popularly cultivated in Thailand, in the Northern provinces of Thailand, particularly in Petchaboon, and the Northeastern Province, Loei. Clinical research shows that curcuma comosa increases the thickness of epithelial cells lining the vaginal canal. The vaginal canal is made up of squamous and stratified epithelial muscles. It is also reported to have aided the repair of vaginal wall prolapse. Vaginal wall prolapse as we discussed in the earlier chapters is a heightened manifestation and symptom of Loose Vagina. Curcuma Comosa therefore is entirely good for tightening vaginal and love muscles. They have been reported to help in relieving vaginal dryness, bad odor, promote circulation to the female genitals, tone saggy muscles and have estrogenic effect. They are said to help make skin glow.

Curcuma Comosa pills may be available in Herbal stores.

BLACKCOHOSH

Black cohosh is a perennial plant that is a member of the buttercup family. Other common names for blackcohosh are: black snakeroot, bugwort, etc. The scientific name for black cohosh is cimicifuga racemosa.

Content and Ingredients in Blackcohosh: Phytochemicals such as beta-carotene, phytosterols, salicylic acid and tannin, calcium, iron, magnesium, phosphorous and B5 vitamin, vitamin A, actaeine, cimicifungin, estrogenic substances, glycosides, isoferulic acid, isoflavones, oleic acid, palmitic acid, racemosin, formononetin, triterpenes, and triterpene saponins. Blackcohosh simulates the effects of estrogen. It may help strengthen the muscles in the pelvic floor, relaxes uterine muscle spasms, thus its suggested use for the treatment of urinary incontinence. It is also used for the treatment of vaginal dryness and hot flashes in menopausal women. In some cases, it has been used to treat depression, anxiety and arthritis. Black cohosh supplements are derived from the roots and underground stems (called rhizomes) of the black cohosh plant. There are suggestions about the potency of the leaves.

PHYTOESTROGENS

Phytoestrogens are plant-based, natural estrogen replacements that provide boost to woman's hormonal levels. Phytoestrogens help to prevent a variety of menopausal symptoms including vaginal dryness. Low estrogen production and levels in the woman body and vaginal dryness are factors in loose vagina. Phytoestrogens are found in foods such as soybeans, soy milk, fermented soy products, tofu, flaxseed, flaxseed oil, and red clover. Phytoestrogens are also present in cherries, legumes, apples, oats, olive oil, garlic, papaya, tomatoes, wheat, pumpkin, sage, fennel, nuts and seeds. Estrogen is also present in eggs. However, the very highest levels of phytoestrogens are found in soy products and also very high in Pueraria mirifica, Mucuna

Pruriens. Peuraria mirifica and Mucuna Prureins are plants found in Asia, and contains interestingly high levels of isoflavones. Pumpkin seeds, flax seeds, rye, and soybeans contain high levels of lignans. Lignans are estrogen-like chemicals which have estrogenic activities in the body system.

BLACK BEANS

Black beans have high levels of magnesium, folate, iron, phosphorous, and muscle building protein. All muscles in the body, including vaginal wall muscles need protein to form and maintain in healthy condition. Protein increases metabolism by helping to build muscle and stall or slow muscle loss that is a natural part of aging. Black beans, and navy beans are full of muscle-building protein: 18 amino acids (with 8 essential amino acids), 19 types of oleic acid, and unsaturated fatty acid. The iron in black beans is very good to prevent iron deficiency anemia which ails most women of child-bearing and menstruating age. When women experience heavy menstrual cycle loss lots of iron in the process and needs replenishment. Iron is good for the making of hemoglobin in the red blood cells. Red blood cells are good in taking nutrients and mainly oxygen to the cells and tissues of the body system, including the cells and tissues of the vaginal wall muscles. **Magnesium** is essential for energy metabolism, proper functioning of the muscle in the body system including vaginal wall muscles and pelvic floor muscles. Magnesium is also good for nerve functions, and formation of cell membranes. Magnesium is also essential in the production of sex hormones like androgen, estrogen and neurotransmitters (dopamine and norepinephrine) that regulates libido. In general, most legumes contain phytoestrogens that are and have about same molecular structure and physiological activity as estrogen and have estrogen-like activity. The said phytoestrogen in legumes help to maintain the hormonal (estrogen) balance in the woman body system. When muscles receive nutrients they require for growth and maintenance, they respond excellently to exercise, and in the case of vaginal wall muscles, they respond well to Kegels.

QUINOA

Quinoa is a native of Andean region of Bolivia, Ecuador, Columbia and Peru. It is a grain-like crop cultivated for its nutrient-rich seeds. It is a pseudo-cereal of the Chenopodium (goosefoot) specie from Chenopodioideae sub-family of the Amarenthaceae family of the animal kingdom. Quinoa contains complete chain of vegetable protein with nine essential amino-acids including omega-3 fatty acids and particularly very high content of lysine. Quinoa is also high in its content of Zinc, B-vitamins, B6, B2, iron, Magnesium, Phosphorous, and Vitamin E. Lysine is the building block/strands of elastin and elastin aids the production of collagen. Elastin is a structural protein responsible for the elastic nature of the connective tissues such as the skin, blood vessels, penis, vaginal walls and canal, Pc muscles, ligaments, lungs, joints, cartilages, etc.

Elastin or otherwise called tropoelastin is a structural protein responsible for elasticity (stretch and recoil) found mainly in connective tissues such as vaginal wall, the penis, skin, blood vessels (chiefly the aorta), joints, ligaments, cartilages. Elastin allows tissue to resume or return to their original shape/size after stretching or contracting. In this case, it helps the vagina to return to its original size after stretches such as in child-birth, insertion of large objects, and loosening and aids the penis to return to its normal size after stretching from excitement. In the human body, elastin is biochemically coded by the gene known as the ELN. Elastin is made up of randomly coiled fibers of about 830 essential amino acids that are cross-linked into a durable form, and lysine is chiefly responsible for the cross-linkage. The two types of links found in elastin are: desmosine link and isodesmosine link. **Remember the ridges or folds of the vaginal wall? Elastin is responsible for the ridges (coils or folds).** Elastin is also found in the bladder and the lungs (expands when full of urine or air respectively and contracts when emptied). Deficiency of elastin may cause diminished elasticity in: Blood vessels: vaginal walls: penile nerves and tissues: and urinary bladder: emphysema (shortness of breath) as in the lungs, caused by alpha-1-antitrypsin deficiency, Marfan's Syndrome. **Elastin** therefore aids in the health of the blood vessels, as such it is very essential to adequate and proper blood circulation and supply. Proper blood circulation and supply is a primer to erection, sexual desire, sexual arousal, sex drive and libido. Elastin maintains the health of the blood vessels surrounding the penis and is the building strands of the vaginal wall muscle fibers. Elastin and collagen works hand in hand and are oftentimes produced simultaneously. Both form the support for the suspension or connecting the vaginal canal to the pelvic floor. And both are replete in the skin around the penis and strands of the penis.

The lysine content of quinoa is high. Lysine, or L-lysine, is an essential amino acid. The human body cannot produce or synthesize lysine. Lysine restores and or promotes the production of arginine in the body system.

Lysine helps restore arginine to its normal levels. L-arginine promotes circulation and relaxes blood vessels. L-arginine is essential for the body production of nitric oxide. Nitric oxide helps to open the potassium channel, which causes the blood vessels to relax – vasodilation, and this aids the proper blood circulation and blood supply to the genitals. Adequate blood supply to the genitals aids sexual arousal, sexual desire, sex drive, and libido. The body system produces its own L-arginine. However, L-lysine aids the arginine to reach its adequate and or optimum level in the body system. **L-arginine** may also stimulate growth hormones and sex hormones, including testosterone which is the libido hormone.

The Zinc in quinoa is good for the production of testosterone, the sex hormone that boosts sexual desire, sexual arousal, sex drive and libido in both men and women. Zinc in combination with B vitamins is excellent for sperm count and fertility. Healthy zinc level in the body is same as healthy testosterone level in the body. Healthy testosterone level in the body (male and female) means high sex drive or high libido. **Iron** in quinoa is good for the formation of new blood cells. Adequate formation of blood cells aid circulation and nutrients are easily taken to destinations and in this case to the genitals. Red blood cells are good for transporting oxygen to the cells of the body including the tissues of the genitals. Adequate supply of oxygen is dependent on healthy blood platelets and in turn dependent on iron supply to the body blood system.

The B-vitamins in quinoa: Vitamin B6 in quinoa helps the body to produce and secrete testosterone, testosterone is excellent for sex drive. This also helps to maintain general hormonal balance. Zinc in combination with B6 raises sperm production, motility, sperm quality/quantity (sperm count or heavy cum) and testosterone production. Low levels of zinc in the body system have been since linked to poor libido in men and women. **Magnesium** in quinoa is good for nerve functions, and formation of cell membranes. Magnesium is also essential in the production of sex hormones like androgen, estrogen and neurotransmitters (dopamine and norepinephrine) that regulates libido. Magnesium helps dilate blood vessels. Vaso-dilation improves blood circulation including the supply of blood to the genitals. Better blood flow to the genitals, creates greater arousal for men and women. Adequate blood supply to the genitals is good for sexual desire and sexual arousal.

Add more quinoa to your diet, for sexual health benefits including sex hormone production and balance, sexual desire, sexual arousal, sex drive and libido. A healthy sex drive and good hormonal balance is a complete precursor to vaginal health including vaginal lubrication and elasticity.

HEALTHY FATS

Healthy fatty acids including omega-3 fatty acids are proven to help for vaginal muscle health and general vaginal wellbeing. Healthy fatty acids are highly present in fishes such as salmon, mackerel, herring, smelts and tuna. It is important to note that most of big fishes may contain high levels of mercury which is not good for health; therefore, you must examine the source of the fishes you are consuming. Smaller fish may be safer in that they often contain insignificant levels of mercury.Omega-3 fatty acids are also found in avocados, flaxseeds, flaxseed oil, borage oil, evening primrose oil and olive oil. Consuming these fishes, and seeds, nuts and some fats and the oils that are high in vitamin E may alleviate problems associated with menopause, atrophic vaginitis, vaginal dryness and loose vagina.

GINSENG: Consuming Ginseng has been said to have positive effects on female hormonal levels. This helps in toning and healthful maintenance of vaginal wall muscles. Consuming ginseng greatly reduces vaginal dryness and pain from intercourse. The active ingredient in Ginseng is gensinosides. Ginseng is known to possess phytoestrogens.

DAMIANA OR WILD YAM (EXTRACT)

The scientific name for the general yam family is Dioscareaceae. The scientific name for Damiana or wild yam is Turnera diffusa. Damiana or wild yam grows in Mexico, Central America and West Africa. In West Africa some varieties of the yam are domestic and is called *"Ji Abana"* and another is wild and called "*Ji Nmuo*" in Igbo language (Eastern Nigeria), and yet another domestic variety is called "*Ji*". They are all very potent and occur in different sizes and colors including colors such as yellow, yellowish green, white and reddish-brown. Wild yam is used in treating impotence. Damiana or wild yam helps to maintain hormonal balance in the body system and also has mildly stimulating properties. Yam contains significant levels of magnesium. It also has high levels of *diosgenin – a steroidal ponins*, which has impact on hormonal pattern and balance. Wild yam extract may help in the treatment of vaginal dryness and other symptoms of menopause.

Asian, oriental, Central American herbalists and naturopathic doctors have recommended wild yam extract for centuries in the treatment of a variety of menstrual and vaginal symptoms. Consuming wild yam and yellow yam have also been said to be very helpful in treating vaginal dryness. **The Steroid Diosgenin**, a steroid sapogenin is extracted from yam including the West African yam, mainly from the species of Dioscorea, such as Dioscorea nipponica. Diosgenin is used for the synthesis (commercial) of progesterone, cortisone, and pregnenolone and some other steroids. The manufactured steroids such as progesterone are then used in some contraceptive pills. Unmodified steroids as found in yams are useful phytochemicals that have estrogenic activities in the body system. They act mainly by reducing the amount of cholesterol in the blood stream thereby regulating the synthesis of estrogen and binding of estrogen to the estrogen receptors. This is a good reason for the use of yam in and as phytoestrogen for regulating estrogen levels in the body. Consuming yam in its natural form therefore is good.

DONG QUAI (ANGELICA SINENSIS)

Angelica sinensis, commonly known as Dong quai is herb from the Apiaceae family of the plant kingdom. The plant is a native of china. Dong quai is <u>not good for pregnant women</u> because it may increase the risk of miscarriage. It is best used by premenstrual and menopausal women.

Dong Quai is an aromatic herb and an oriental herb that grows abundantly in China, Korea, and Japan. Herbalists use Dong Quai in the treatment of a variety of gynecological complications including vaginal dryness, painful sexual intercourse, and regulation of menstrual as well as menopausal problems.

Dong Quai contains vitamin E, B12, and A. It is also very rich in tannins and tannic acid. Other phytochemicals in the herb includes coumarins, phytosterols, polysaccharides, ferulate, and flavonoids. It also has analgesic, sedative and anti-inflammatory properties. It may also reduce blood pressure and fatigue.

EPINEDIUM SAGITTATUM (HORNY GOAT WEED)

The horny goat weed herb is mainly found in Asia and the Mediterranean. The Chinese call it Yin Yang Huo, and it means "sexy goat plant" There are various species and varieties of the plant.

However, all the specie contains the active ingredient (icariin) to a different degree. Horny goat weed is known to have other sexual health and general health benefits. However, its enlistment for the health of the vagina muscles is based on the fact that it helps blood circulation and blood supply to the genitals, encouraging lasting erection and engorgement of the female genitals. Icariin is a phytoestrogen and works by blocking the activity of a particular enzyme in the body, with similar effect of some prescription drugs that treat erectile dysfunction. Healthy blood supply to the genitals means supply of nutrients to the cells, tissues and muscles of the genitals including vaginal wall muscles. Furthermore, some flavonoids in some species of horny goat weed have flavonoid with potent and specific estrogen receptor (ER) bioactivity. Studies in laboratory animals show that horny goat weed may influence levels of neurotransmitters such as norepinephrine, serotonin, and dopamine and reduce cortisol levels. The herb/leaves of horny goat weed may be used frequently; however, the supplement is better used on an intermittent basis. The herbal supplement may be available from drug and herbal stores.

TRIBULUS TERRESTRIS

Tribulus terrestris is mainly found in China and South Africa. In china, it is a traditional herb. It's used to enhance sexual function, increase muscle mass, alleviates urinary incontinence, and improve sperm motility. Some mixtures of different compounds (phytochemicals) found in the fruits, stems and roots of the plant - tribulus terrestris provide its medicinal properties. It's said that such phytochemicals present in tribulus terrestris may encourage increase in the body levels of hormones such as testosterone and dehydroepiandrosterone, or DHEA. Testosterone helps to maintain estrogen balance in the body system, DHEA is converted to estrogen in body and maintains estrogen balance which is essential to reduces vaginal dryness, and curing atrophic vaginitis – proud symptoms of loose vagina. Good testosterone level in the body improves the time the body muscles needs to recover from any health lapse and enhances protein synthesis using the body's constituent amino acids. Normal testosterone level also promotes positive estrogen balance. The combination of these actions all help to strengthen and increase the body muscle mass, including vaginal wall muscle. The only side effects that may be experienced include upset stomach, which can be helped/reduced/eliminated if the herb/supplement is taken with food. The herbal supplement may be available from drug and herbal stores.

HYPOTHETICAL SIDE EFFECT OF TRIBULUS

However, caution need be exercised here by **pregnant women and breast-feeding mothers**. Considering that, as explained herein, tribulus terrestris increases testosterone level, it then means that the possibility of side effects may include anger and rage, lowering of the female voice, increased body or facial hair, increase in the size of or an enlarged prostate or the worsening of hormone-related cancer such as breast or prostate cancer.

OTHER FOODS WITH ESTROGEN AND ESTROGEN-LIKE PHYTOCHEMICALS: -

LIQOURICE

Liquorice is the root of the plant <u>Glycyrrhiza glabra</u>. It is a legume, and the sweet taste is driven from the active ingredient/compound glycyrrhizin (a natural sweetener) and the flavor comes from the compound anethole. It is called Athimathuram in Tamil. In Sanskrit, it is called Yashtimadhu and in Northern India it is called Mulethi. Liquorice flavor is found in a range of liquorice candies reinforced by anise seed oil, tarragon oil or fennel oil because they have similar flavor. The stick and root can be chew and are available in sweet shops and some herbal shops. Liquorice root induces the production of estrogen, which is essential for sexual functioning. A good level of the hormone estrogen in the woman body system is essential to maintain vaginal health. The active ingredient in liquorice (glycyrrhezenic acid) affects the body's endocrine system. The effect on the endocrine system is because of the isoflavones (Phytoestrogen) content of the gycyrrhezenic acid. The effect reduces the blood level of testosterone, and in so doing help in maintaining hormonal balance mainly beneficial to women. Consuming liquorice candy in excess may be toxic to the liver, the cardiovascular system and may produce hypertension and edema swelling from accumulation of fluid under the skin).

MACA ROOT

The scientific name for Maca Root is Lepidium Meyenii. It is native to South America and particularly to the Andes and the

Inca natives of Peru, and Bolivia. Maca Root is very rich in selenium, calcium, magnesium and iron, amino acids and fatty acids. It helps in producing and maintaining good levels of sex drive and libido which induces vaginal lubrication warding off dryness.

FENNEL

Fennel is rich in estrogen and estrogen-like substance. Fennel may be libido-enhancing.

GARLIC

Garlic contains an active ingredient called allicin, which boosts circulation and blood flow to sexual organs. When the sexual organs including the vaginal walls and the pelvic floor are proper supplied with blood, they are supplied with nutrients. The vaginal wall muscles need proper nutrients for proper functioning.

GINGER

Ginger root stimulates circulation and increases blood flow to the vital sex organs, including the vaginal walls, the pelvic floor and the vulva. A well blood-circulated vaginal wall muscle is invariably supplied with nutrients.

HESPERIDIN

Hesperidin is a citrus bioflavonoid. Contents of Hesperin include the flavonoid - flavonne glycoside (glucoside), the flavonne hesperitin, and deschloride rutinose.

Hesperin is very predominant in lemons and peppers. Hesperin is most abundant and concentrated in the rinds and peel of oranges, peppers, lemons and tangerine. Orange juice with pulp has more flavonoids than orange juice without pulp. The combination of vitamin C, rutin and hesperin as found in the said sources is an excellent combination for the health and rejuvenation of epithelial and connective tissues and cells as found in the vaginal wall and the pelvic floor. Hesperidin and a flavonne glycoside diosmin are used to treat and support the health of veins, venous insufficiency and hemorrhoids. Hesperidin is said to be helpful in maintaining capillary health, thus improving circulation and supply of nutrients to epithelial cells and tissues. Hesperidin may also have anti-inflammatory effects. Because of its assistance in maintaining capillary health, it is said to be very useful in treating vericose veins and bruising. It also works in combination with Vitamin C to maintain the health of collagen lining of the vaginal canal. Collagen and elastin form part of support for the attachment of the vagina to the pelvic floor.

WHEAT GERM

Wheat germ contains lots of Vitamin E and omega-3 fatty acids. Vitamin E helps the body to synthesize sex hormones. Vitamin E also helps the woman's body system hormonal (estrogen) balance. When a woman's estrogen is in balance, it is in optimum level. Estrogen adequacy helps to reduce vaginal dryness, atrophic vaginitis, and loose vagina. A woman with a balance estrogen level also experience less premenstrual stress (PMS), less anxiety, headaches and mood swings, invariably her sex drive may improve.

CAVIAR (ROE or FISH EGGS)

Eggs harvested from most notably unfertilized sturgeon and salmon. There are red and black caviar. Roe or fish eggs could be harvested from Beluga Sturgeon, Sevruga or Stellate Sturgeon, Dog Salmon, Pink Salmon. Beluga is the largest of sturgeon fishes with the largest caviar. Caviar contains nutrients such as: selenium, iron, magnesium, calcium and phosphorus, phospholipids and omega-3 fatty acids, omega-6 fatty acids, potassium, vitamin D, vitamin A, vitamin E. **Selenium** in caviar is vital to ensure the production of healthy ova & sperms. It acts as a coenzyme to calcium and magnesium. **Magnesium** in caviar is essential for energy metabolism, proper functioning of the muscle in the body system including vaginal wall muscles and pelvic floor muscles. Magnesium is also good for nerve functions, and formation of cell membranes. Magnesium is also essential in the production of sex hormones like androgen, estrogen and neurotransmitters (dopamine and norepinephrine) that regulates libido. Deficiency of magnesium in the body may lead to muscle weakness, irregular heartbeat, muscle spasms or twitches. Magnesium is good for energy metabolism and protein synthesis.

Calcium in caviar is essential for the growth, maintenance and reproduction processes of the human body. Calcium is mainly known for its functions to maintain strong healthy bones and teeth of the body and for the prevention of the onset of osteoporosis. The attention catching property of calcium in caviar is the help it gives to the normal muscle contraction and relaxation cycle and its help in hormonal secretion. **Phosphorous** in caviar is required by nearly every cell and tissue of the body for optimal functioning. This is also very helpful, noting that deficiency in the body level of phosphorous may lead to muscle weakness, and anemia. **Potassium** in caviar plays a role in metabolism and body functions such as acid-base regulation, muscle and body growth. It aids the muscle contraction and relaxation. It helps general muscle health. **Healthy fatty acids** including omega-3 and omega-6 fatty acids are proven help for vaginal muscle health and general vaginal wellbeing.

Vitamin E in caviar helps the body to synthesize sex hormones. Vitamin E also helps the woman's body system hormonal (estrogen) balance. When a woman's estrogen is in balance, it is in optimum level. Estrogen adequacy helps to reduce vaginal dryness, atrophic vaginitis, and loose vagina. A woman with a balance estrogen level also experience less premenstrual stress (PMS), less anxiety, headaches and mood swings, invariably her sex drive may improve.

Vitamin A in caviar helps to maintain the health of the epithelial tissues which line all the external and internal surfaces of the body, including the linings of the vaginal wall and the uterus in women. Vaginal wall consists of stratified squamous epithelial muscles. Generally, sex hormones including estrogen have DNA receptor sites, and vitamin A is in the family that is friendly to the receptors.

Vitamin A in caviar helps the regulation of the synthesis of the sex hormone, progesterone, which in turn helps in balancing the levels of estrogen. Vitamin A has a direct activity towards the regulation of sexual growth, development, and reproduction by turning and switching on genes in response to sex hormone triggers. Vitamin A can also increase hormonal (progesterone) development. Progesterone is associated with improved sexual urge and the power to remain active for a longer time. **Vitamin D** in caviar is an essential part of the endocrine system. Vitamin D helps to regulate several of the adrenal hormones, growth of cells, and production of enzymes. **DHEA** is produced by the adrenal glands. DHEA or Dehydroepiandrosterone is a steroid hormone produced by the body to create both male and female hormones. DHEA is secreted naturally in the body by the adrenal glands. DHEA and estrogen hormone levels in the body tends to peak in the twenties and decline as people get older. DHEA is converted in the body to both the female hormone, estrogen and the male hormone testosterone.

KELP/ALGAE/SEAWEED

Kelp or algae extract is derived from seaweed. Kelp, a seaweed is a rich source of iodine, calcium, zinc, magnesium, selenium and iron, Vitamin B9 -folate, Vitamins A and K, and amino acids – L-Lysine. Calcium in kelp is essential for the growth, maintenance and reproduction processes of the human body. Calcium is mainly known for its functions to maintain strong healthy bones and teeth of the body and for the prevention of the onset of osteoporosis. The attention catching property of calcium in kelp is the help it gives to the normal muscle contraction and relaxation cycle and its help in hormonal secretion.

Selenium in kelp is vital to ensure the production of healthy ova & sperms. It acts as a coenzyme to calcium and magnesium. Magnesium in kelp is essential for energy metabolism, proper functioning of the muscle in the body system including vaginal wall muscles and pelvic floor muscles. Magnesium is also good for nerve functions, and formation of cell membranes. Magnesium is also essential in the production of sex hormones like androgen, estrogen and neurotransmitters (dopamine and norepinephrine) that regulates libido. Deficiency of magnesium in the body may lead to muscle weakness, irregular heartbeat, muscle spasms or twitches. Magnesium is good for energy metabolism and protein synthesis. The iron in kelp is very good to prevent iron deficiency anemia which ails most women of child-bearing and menstruating age. When women experience heavy menstrual cycle loss lots of iron in the process and needs replenishment. Iron is good for the making of hemoglobin in the red blood cells. Red blood cells are good in taking nutrients and mainly oxygen to the cells and tissues of the body system, including the cells and tissues of the vaginal wall muscles. **Vitamin A** in kelp helps the regulation of the synthesis of the sex hormone, progesterone, which in turn helps in balancing the levels of estrogen. Vitamin A has a direct activity towards the regulation of sexual growth, development, and reproduction by turning and switching on genes in response to sex hormone triggers. Vitamin A can also increase hormonal (progesterone) development. Progesterone is associated with improved sexual urge and the power to remain active for a longer time.

BORON FOOD SOURCES: -

Prunes, Hazelnuts, Peanuts, Kiwi, Plum, Pear

All of the above contain reasonable amounts of boron. Boron is a trace mineral/element. Boron increases levels of estrogen in women and testosterone in men. It is used to help regulate sex hormones, especially in women going through menopause, and diminishes the need for Hormone replacement therapy (HRT). Boron regimen in premenopausal, menopausal and postmenopausal women presents fast result in improved sex drive, libido and vaginal lubrication. Symptom of menopause such as hot flashes and depression were quickly eliminated in women undergoing boron regimen. Adequate levels of boron are required for healthy mental function. Boron is good to ward off depression and memory loss. Depression leads to low sex drive/low libido, and associated dryness. Boron plays an important role in maintaining trans-membrane functions and in stabilizing the hormone reception. Boron is essential for the metabolism of minerals such as calcium, magnesium and copper. Foods rich in boron are almonds, prunes, avocados and hazelnuts. Other sources of Boron are Kiwi, red grapes, dates, pear, plum, onion, pea nuts butter, lentil, etc. Boron is good and has shown success in the treatment of arthritis and rheumatoid arthritis. Dietary sources of boron are excellent. However, one can overdose on supplemental boron. Boron could become toxic in high doses, use with care.

PECAN

Pecans are a good source of protein and both monounsaturated and polyunsaturated fats including L-arginine. Pecan is also very rich source of manganese, magnesium, phosphorous, zinc, thiamine, and Iron. L-arginine in pecan helps to stimulate the release of growth hormone (GH), dopamine and other substances into the body system. Growth hormones and dopamine help in the production of testosterone which is essential for sexual desire, sexual arousal, and vaginal lubrication. L-arginine induces the release of nitric oxide in the body. Nitric acid relaxes the arteries, reducing the pressure on the arteries, reducing blood vessels stiffness and encourages optimal flow and circulation of blood. In so doing, nitric oxide aids the supply of adequate nutrients to the genitals, thus encouraging the genital and encouraging vaginal lubrication. This is also good for the female libido by aiding blood flow to the genitals. Blood engorgement of the female sex organ is a primer for sexual desire, sexual arousal, sex drive and libido. **Magnesium** in pecan is essential for energy metabolism, proper functioning of the muscle in the body system including vaginal wall muscles and pelvic floor muscles. Magnesium is also good for nerve functions, and formation of cell membranes. Magnesium is also essential in the production of sex hormones like androgen, estrogen and neurotransmitters (dopamine and norepinephrine) that regulates libido. Magnesium helps dilate blood vessels. Vaso-dilation improves blood circulation including the supply of blood to the genitals. Better blood flow to the genitals, creates greater arousal for men and women.

Adequate blood supply to the genitals is good for sexual desire, sexual arousal and vaginal lubrication. **The Zinc** in pecan is good for the production of testosterone, the sex hormone that boosts sexual desire, sexual arousal, sex drive and libido in both men and women. Healthy zinc level in the body is same as healthy testosterone level in the body. Healthy testosterone level in the body (male and female) means high sex drive or high libido. **Manganese** in pecan is essential for the synthesis of fatty acids, which is necessary for a healthy nervous system. The nervous system is the electrical system of the body.

Vitamin E is the sex, reproductive and fertility vitamin. **Iron** in pecan is good for the making of hemoglobin in the red blood cells. Iron is mainly lost or wasted from the body system during menstruation. Red blood cells are good in taking nutrients and mainly oxygen to the cells and tissues of the body system, including the cells and tissues of the genitals. Daily consumption of pecans may delay age-related muscle nerve degeneration, and muscle wasting or losing, including vaginal muscles. **Extra info - FYI**: A diet rich in nuts can lower the risk of gallstone in women. The antioxidants and phytosterols present in pecans reduce high cholesterol by eliminating the LDL (bad Cholesterol) while preserving the HDL (good cholesterol). Daily consumption of a handful of pecans may help lower cholesterol (LDL) levels just the same way the marketed cholesterol lowering medication do. It is good to know that most of the so-called cholesterol lowering medications are extracted phytosterols (plant sterols) marketed as cytellin. Daily consumption of pecans may delay age-related muscle nerve degeneration, and muscle wasting or losing, including vaginal muscles.

NUTMEG

Elemicin, an active ingredient in Nutmeg is a neuromuscular blocker and could be useful in treating urinary incontinence. Nutmeg is the roughly egg-shaped seed of the Nutmeg tree. The nutmeg tree is of the genus Myristica. The common or fragrant nutmeg tree, *Myristica fragrans*, is a native of the Banda Islands of Indonesia. It is also grown in Penang Island of Malaysia, the Caribbean and Grenada. The active ingredients in the seed of the nutmeg are: Elemicin, and Myristicin. Large dose of raw and freshly ground nutmeg produces psychoactive, hallucinations and euphoric effects on users. **Elemicin** is a phenylpropene (a natural organic anticholinergenic compound) and causes an anticholinergic-like effect on a person. As an anticholinergenic, elemicin blocks the action of the neurotransmitter acetylcholine in both the Central Nervous System (CNS – Brain + Spinal cord) and the Peripheral Nervous system (blood vessels and nerves besides brain and spinal cord) from binding to its receptor nerves cells/fibers. The nerve fibers of the parasympathetic system are responsible for the involuntary movements of smooth muscles present in body such as: Urinary tract/bladder, pelvic floor muscles, genital muscles, lungs, etc. During intercourse and orgasm, the smooth muscles of the genitals contracts involuntarily for orgasm to happen. The anticholinergenic effect of elemicin prolongs and helps you to control the contraction of the PC/genital muscles. Nutmeg's elemicin is a neuromuscular blocker and could be useful in treating urinary incontinence. Anticholinergenics are divided into three categories to represent their targets in the central and/or peripheral nervous system: antimuscarinic agents, ganglionic blockers, and neuromuscular blockers. Other examples of anticholinergenics include: atropine and dicycloverine. Myristicin belongs to the class of monoamine oxidase inhibitors (MAOIs). Monoamine oxidase inhibitors are a class of antidepressant drugs, used in the treatment of atypical/unusual/light depression. This is what provides the euphoria from nutmeg.

Myristicin is responsible for the euphoria and the hallucination.

****

CAUTION!

The following vegetables of the cruciferous family (mainly Broccoli) though are very healthy, being rich in Vitamin K, Vitamin C, magnesium, folate, and Vitamin E and are sex drive and libido booster mainly in men; however, they have been proven to contain indole-3-carbinol. Indole-3-carbinol is well-known for its anti-estrogenic effects, estrogen reducer. Indole-3-carbinol is used to treat estrogen dominance (excessive estrogen) in both men and women. Caution must be exercised when enlisting indole-3-carbinol rich foods and vegetables, except in situations of estrogen dominance. Occurrence of excessive estrogen is very unlikely in premenopausal,

menopausal women. It is not yet very clear if Indole-3-carbinol in these cruciferous vegetables activates only when the body levels of estrogen is already high enough to make it active.

****

Vegetable of the cruciferous family listed below are potent sources of magnesium, which helps dilate blood vessels. Vaso-dilation improves blood circulation including the supply of blood to the genitals. Better blood flow to the genitals, creates greater arousal for men and women. Adequate blood supply to the genitals is good for sexual desire and sexual arousal.

However, members of the cruciferous vegetable family have been shown to contain indole-3-carbinol. Indole-3-carbinol decreases the level of estrogen in the male body system – **good for the man.** This is achieved by indole-3-carbinol adhering to the estrogen nerve end receptors thus preventing the binding of excess estrogen to the receptors. In so doing it helps to prevent estrogen dominance in both male and female, thus promoting hormonal balance and optimal level of testosterone which is a potent primer of sex drive and libido. Indole-3-carbinol has been shown to be beneficial in treating Lupus. Lupus is associated with estrogen, sometimes called estrogen disease. Indole-3-carbinol induces DNA repair in cells and inhibits the growth of cancer cells. Broccoli consumption is good for prostate health. Consumption of broccoli may also cause malodorous flatulence. Cruciferous vegetables can be metabolized to sulforaphane, an anti-cancer compound. Spinach and other green cruciferous vegetables including:

- ✓ Broccoli
- ✓ Spinach
- ✓ Brussels sprouts
- ✓ Kale
- ✓ Cabbage,
- ✓ Swiss chard
- ✓ Bok Choy

They are also good sources of magnesium and folate. Folate (vitamin B9) is a good vitamin for fertility and reproductive health. Folate may also lower blood levels of a harmful substance called homocysteine. Homocysteine is an amino acid, that is very unfriendly to the lining of arteries and encourages plaque adhere and accumulate on the walls of arteries, increasing the risk of peripheral arterial disease (PAD). Magnesium, folic acid, Vitamin C, Vitamin K, Vitamin E are abundant in other food sources and also as supplements from health stores.

BF

CHAPTER 6

- ❖ **VITAMINS**
- ❖ **SUPPLEMENTS**
- ❖ **MINERALS**
- ❖ **GRADE OILS**

FOR VAGINAL TIGHTENING

Vitamins provide substances that a woman's body may not be producing due to hormonal imbalance and other nutritional deficiencies.

VITAMIN E

Vitamin E has been said to aid in the production of sex hormones including estrogen.

Vitamin E oil sometimes called the sex vitamin is helpful for rejuvenating dry vaginal tissues when taken orally and when used as a topical application. You can get vitamin E from your diet, however, dietary vitamin E may not provide a large enough quantity to supply your body with what you need to overcome vaginal dryness. In this light, you may want to take an oral and topical vitamin E oil supplement to aid in relieving your vaginal dryness and vaginal tightness. Taking doses of the vitamin, say 400 to 800 IU daily, may help a woman's body produce estriol and progesterone to maintain estrogen balance. Vitamin E is also important for women going through the premenopausal phase. In general, perimenopause usually start between ages 45 and 49. Almost all symptoms of sex drive and vaginal health in this phase of a woman's life is caused by wild fluctuation in estrogen levels. Vitamin E helps the body conserve the building blocks of estrogen, estriol, and the progesterone it needs for hormonal balance.

Vitamin E aids the supply of nutrients and oxygen to the sex organs by encouraging circulation and supply of blood to the sex organ. Vitamin E also helps to protect the ova from damage. Vitamin E in combination with zinc are good for the body to attain proper functioning of the sex organs including the vagina, vulva, pelvic floor and vaginal wall muscles.

TOPICAL APPLICATION OF VITAMIN E OIL

The topical application of vitamin E oil is mainly for lubrication. Some women use the oil from Vitamin E capsules to replicate vaginal lubrication. Applying Vitamin E oil on a daily basis rehydrates the vaginal tissues. The walls of the vaginal canal incorporate the moisture from vitamin E oil back into its natural processes. Remember the vaginal wall oozes out moisture into the canal during arousal and intercourse. The Vitamin E can be used episodically as a lubricant before intercourse.

The use of all-natural vitamin E oil is far better and healthier to use in lubricating the vaginal canal and walls than the over-the-counter lubricants because the over-the-counter vaginal lubricants contains drying chemicals or scents. Use vitamin E oil instead of vaginal lubricants. Vitamin E oil is high in nutrients that nourish the vaginal wall and vaginal muscles. As the vaginal walls absorb the nutrients in vitamin E oil, it heals and alleviates the problems associated with perimenopause, menopause, atrophic vaginitis, vaginal dryness and loose vagina. Insert a 600 IU to 800 UI vitamin E gel cap into the vagina at bedtime for relief of dryness. As the gel capsule dissolves the vitamin E oil coats and lubricates vaginal tissues. You may also insert another capsule of vitamin E oil into the vagina as you set off for work. Vitamin E oil is available at health food stores and in most drug stores. Far from the oil of the vitamin E capsule, the capsule itself is mainly made of Gelatin. Gelatin is hydrolyzed collagen and elastin. The vaginal muscles are lined/made-up of collagen and elastin. Elastin is responsible for the folds and coils of the vaginal walls inside the vaginal canal, which is responsible for the elasticity of the vagina. Elastin is also responsible for penile erection (stretching) and recoil. The gelatin dissolves and some may be absorbed and incorporated into the vaginal wall. Elastin and Collagen are both structural proteins and are together responsible for vaginal elasticity and tightness/firmness.

VITAMIN A

Vitamin A maintains the health of the epithelial tissues which line all the external and internal surfaces of the body, including the linings of the vagina wall and the uterus in women. Vaginal wall consists of stratified squamous epithelial muscles.

Generally, sex hormones including estrogen have DNA receptor sites, and vitamin A is in the family that is friendly to the receptors. Vitamin A helps in the regulation of the synthesis of the sex hormone, progesterone, which in turn helps in balancing the levels of estrogen. Vitamin A has a direct activity towards the regulation of sexual growth, development, and reproduction by turning and switching on genes in response to sex hormone triggers. Vitamin A can also increase hormonal (progesterone) development. Progesterone is associated with improved sexual urge and the power to remain active for a longer time.

BETACAROTENE

Beta-carotene capsules/supplement may also be used in place of Vitamin A. Beta-carotene is converted to vitamin A in the body system and one can never overdose on beta-carotene, nor can the body reach any toxic level of beta-carotene. The conversion of beta-carotene to vitamin A is only done as and when the body needs it. Do not use Beta-carotene and Vitamin A at the same time. It is one or the other, and not together. Carrot is very rich in beta-carotene.

ELASTIN

Elastin or otherwise called tropoelastin is a structural protein found mainly in connective tissues such as vaginal wall, penile tissues (penis), skin, blood vessels (chiefly the aorta), joints. Elastin allows tissue to resume or return to their original shape/size after stretching or contracting. In this case, it helps the vagina to return to its original size after stretches such as in child-birth, insertion of large objects, and loosening. In the human body, elastin is biochemically coded by the gene known as the ELN.

Elastin is made up of randomly coiled fibers of about 830 essential amino acids that are cross-linked into a durable form, and lysine is chiefly responsible for the cross-linkage. The two types of links found in elastin are: desmosine link and isodesmosine link.

Remember the ridges or folds of the vaginal wall? Elastin is responsible for the ridges (coils or folds). Elastin is also found in the bladder and the lungs (expands when full of urine or air respectively and contracts when emptied). Deficiency of elastin causes: General loss of elasticity such as in Loose vagina, Loose bladder (incontinence), in-erectable penis, emphysema (shortness of breath) as in the lungs, caused by alpha-1-antitrypsin deficiency. Marfan's Syndrome

Food Sources of Elastin includes:

Plant sources – Beans, lentils, soy, legumes, pea, amaranth, maize or corn /cornmeal for containing lysine, proline, glycine, alanine, and valine.

Animal sources – Bovine, Chicken, Poultry, Pork, non-fat milk, beef, eggs, parmesan cheese

Sea food Sources – fatty fishes, sardine, salmon, caviar, catfish Gelatin (hydrolyzed collagen).

SUPPLEMENT Forms

Elastin, Lysine, Alanine, Proline, Valine, Glycine, Allysin.

COLLAGEN

Collagen like elastin is commonly found in penile tissues, vaginal muscles, connective tissues such as ligaments, blood vessels, skin, bones, eye(cornea) and gut in the form of elongated fibril (strands of fibrillin -glycoproteins).

Collagen is created in the body cells called fibroblast. In muscle tissue, it serves as a major component of the endomysium. The endomysium is a layer that covers/en-sheaths the muscle fiber made-up of mostly reticular fibers.

There are 28 types of known collagen including:

Type I Collagen - commonly found in the Skin, organs, tendon, vascular ligature, and bone

Type II Collagen – commonly found in the cartilage

Type III Collagen –commonly found in reticular fibers alongside type1

Type IV Collagen – commonly found in cell base membrane

Type V Collagen – commonly found on cell surfaces, hair, hair follicular base and placenta

Over 90% of the collagen in the body, however, is of type one.

Stress (cortisol) causes the degradation of skin collagen to amino acids. Type I and Type III collagen are mainly used and imparted during reconstructive surgery, as artificial substitutes. Why surgery when you can take the substance as supplement and avoid the risks associated with surgery.

SUPPLEMENT Forms

Type I Collagen and Type II Collagen are supplementary collagen for vaginal tightening.

However, collagen is a protein and proteins must be metabolized (broken down) into constituent amino acids before absorption, amino acids supplements may offer quicker absorption.

Amino Acid Supplements include: lysine, proline, glycine, alanine, and valine.

FOOD SOURCES of Collagen/Amino Acids

Plant sources – Beans, lentils, soy, legumes, pea, amaranth, maize or corn /cornmeal for containing lysine, proline, glycine, alanine, and valine. **Animal sources** –Bovine, Chicken, Poultry, Pork, non-fat milk, beef, eggs, parmesan cheese **Sea Food Sources** – fatty fishes, sardine, salmon, caviar, catfish, Gelatin (hydrolyzed collagen)

DHEA

DHEA or Dehydroepiandrosterone is a steroid substance produced by the body to create both male and female hormones. DHEA itself is neither a hormone nor a vitamin; however, it is a precursor, aid, primer and or regulator of sex hormones. DHEA is secreted naturally in the body by the adrenal glands. DHEA and estrogen hormone levels in the body tends to peak in the twenties and decline as people get older. DHEA is converted in the body to both the female hormone, estrogen and the male hormone testosterone. Levels of DHEA decline naturally with age and this can lead to decreased estrogen levels and subsequently atrophic vaginitis, vaginal dryness, vaginal itching, decreased sex drive, decreased libido and ultimately loose vagina. DHEA is available over the counter in most drug stores in USA. However, it is good to remember that hormones are precision substances in that at any point, hormones require the proper balance to work effectively. And when you overdose on them, the resulting imbalance may cause health problems rather than improve them. You are therefore advised to consult an experienced professional before employing hormonal replacement therapy and make sure you have the correct dosage and are in good health. DHEA is neither a hormone nor a vitamin, however, it plays a vital role in hormonal production, regulation and balance. Intermittent (off-on) use of this precursor may be safe.

VITAMIN C

Vitamin C is involved in the synthesis of sex hormones such as androgen, estrogen and progesterone. Vitamin C helps to increase libido and also highly effective in increasing fertility. Vitamin C is essential for the production of collagen and elastin, both forms part of the support to the vaginal attachment to the pelvic floor. Elastin is the structural protein responsible for the elasticity of the vagina, the vaginal wall and vaginal canal.

VITAMIN D

Vitamin D is an essential part of the endocrine system. Vitamin D helps to regulate several of the adrenal hormones, growth of cells, and production of enzymes. DHEA is produced by the adrenal glands. DHEA or Dehydroepiandrosterone is a steroid hormone produced by the body to create both male and female hormones. DHEA is secreted naturally in the body by the adrenal glands. DHEA and estrogen hormone levels in the body tends to peak in the twenties and decline as people get older. DHEA is converted in the body to both the female hormone, estrogen and the male hormone testosterone.

VITAMIN B6

Vitamin B6 is necessary for metabolism of protein, fat and amino acids, hormonal function (estrogen and testosterone), and the production of red blood cells, and neurotransmitters-

(serotonin, norepinephrine, dopamine, GABA –gama-aminobutyric acid). GABA is directly responsible for the regulation of muscle tone including smooth muscles such as vaginal and pc muscles. Vitamin B6 is essential for the general good of the nervous system. **It is very important for keeping stress away**. Vitamin B6 is directly involved in synthesis and secretion of dopamine in the brain. Dopamine gives a feel-good mood. Feel-good mood is love mood and sex drive friendly. Vitamin B6 is essential for conversion of selenium in its dietary state (selenomethionine) into an absorbable form by the body. Vitamin B6 helps in controlling elevated prolactin and in so doing functions as a libido enhancer. Vitamin B6 helps to balance the levels of progesterone and estrogen. Ingesting Vitamin B6 regularly, helps a woman reach orgasm and sometimes increases sexual stamina.

VITAMIN B12 + VITAMIN B9

Vitamin B12 may help in improving vaginal dryness by regulating and improving the function of adrenal gland. In regulating the adrenal functions, the B vitamins help to regulate the production of DHEA which is converted to estrogen and is essential to the hormonal balance of the body and to vaginal health, vaginal muscle health, alleviate vaginal dryness and restore vaginal elasticity, curing loose vagina by making it tight again. Intake of Vitamin B12 in combination with Vitamin B9 (folic acid), may help the body system to function properly. Vitamin B9 is a good vitamin for fertility and reproductive health. Vitamin B12 is essential to the proper and optimal function of the body system.

The B vitamins are water soluble and as such are not stored in the body quite unlike the fat-soluble vitamins. This means that though the body has a recommended daily value, reaching a toxic level of the B vitamins in the body is not possible, as they could not be stored in the body.

ARGININE OR L-ARGININE

Arginine is an amino acid, also referred to as L-arginine. It is a very popular amino acid and supplements for sexual dysfunction for both men and women. Arginine helps stimulates the body to release growth hormone among other substances and is converted into nitric oxide in the body. Nitric oxide is a compound that helps in the health of blood vessels, improving the flow of adequate blood through the arteries and to the sexual organs, including vaginal wall muscles, PC/love muscles. Adequate blood supply to the vaginal wall muscles means good supply of nutrients to the cells and tissues of the vaginal wall muscles. L-Arginine can be taken in herbal pill form. However, many women interviewed report that they achieved the best results by applying a cream directly where it counts. Foods rich in L-Arginine include granola, oatmeal, peanuts, cashews, walnuts, dairy, green vegetables, root vegetables, garlic, ginseng, soybeans, chickpea, seeds and nuts.

****

MINERALS FOR VAGINAL TIGHTENING

MAGNESIUM

Magnesium is essential for energy metabolism, proper functioning of the muscle in the body system including vaginal wall muscles and pelvic floor muscles.

Magnesium is also good for nerve functions, and formation of cell membranes. Magnesium is also essential in the production of sex hormones like androgen, estrogen and neurotransmitters (dopamine and norepinephrine) that regulates libido. Deficiency of magnesium in the body may lead to muscle weakness, irregular heartbeat, muscle spasms or twitches. Magnesium is good for energy metabolism and protein synthesis.

Magnesium helps dilate blood vessels and as such helps in proper blood circulation to the genitals including the vaginal, vulva and the vaginal wall. Better blood flow to the genitals, creates greater arousal for men and women. Magnesium-rich foods include artichokes, bananas, dried figs, prune juice, yogurt, spinach and potatoes, leafy green vegetables, seaweed or green algae, avocados, nuts, beans, raw chocolate, and grains such as brown rice and millet.

SELENIUM

Selenium is vital to ensure the production of healthy ova & sperms. It acts as a coenzyme to calcium and magnesium. Foods with high selenium content include Brazil nuts, tuna, oysters, celery, orange rinds and wheat flour.

CALCIUM

Calcium is essential for the growth, maintenance and reproduction processes of the human body. Calcium is mainly known for its functions to maintain strong healthy bones and teeth of the body and for the prevention of the onset of osteoporosis. The attention catching property of calcium for consideration for this topic is the help it gives to the normal muscle contraction and relaxation cycle and its help in hormonal secretion.

You can ingest Calcium as a supplement or from your daily diet. Plant sources include green leafy vegetables, kale and broccoli, beans and almonds. Animal sources of calcium include milk, yogurt and cheese

POTASSIUM

Potassium plays a role in metabolism and body functions such as acid-base regulation, muscle and body growth. It aids the muscle contraction and relaxation. It helps general muscle health. Banana is particularly rich in potassium, manganese and magnesium. Other plant food sources rich in potassium include orange juice, vegetables such as sweet potatoes and Irish potatoes (including the back peel), squash, broccoli, and citrus fruits. Animal sources of potassium include red meat, chicken, milk and seafood such as salmon, cod, and tuna.

PHOSPHOROUS

Phosphorous is required by nearly every cell and tissue of the body for optimal functioning. This is also very helpful, noting that deficiency in the body level of phosphorous may lead to muscle weakness, and anemia. Plant sources of phosphorous include almonds and peanuts. Animal food sources are milk, cheese, yogurt, eggs, and beef.

MANGANESE

Manganese is essential for the synthesis of fatty acids, which is necessary for a healthy nervous system. The nervous system is somewhat the electrical system of the body. The nervous system regulates the production and secretion of hormones.

****

CUSMETIC GRADE OILS FOR TREATING VAGINAL DRYNESS

COCONUT OIL

Cosmetic grade (pure) Virgin Coconut oil can be applied directly to the vagina for lubrication and during intercourse to make it less painful and offer more lubrication. Virgin Coconut oil is safe for sensitive vaginal skin. It helps to sooth, rejuvenates and alleviates vaginal dryness. The vaginal wall absorbs the ingredients present in the virgin coconut oil and it aids in healing. Virgin coconut oil is:

- ✓ Odorless
- ✓ Tasteless
- ✓ Inexpensive
- ✓ Soothing

✓ Anti-bacterial

Coconut oil is available from pharmacies, drug stores and high-quality health food stores.

OLIVE OIL

Extra virgin olive oil can be applied directly to the vagina for lubrication and during intercourse to make it less painful and offer more lubrication. Extra virgin olive oil is safe for sensitive vaginal skin. It helps to sooth, rejuvenates and alleviates vaginal dryness. Extra virgin olive oil contains vitamin E, omega-3 fatty acids; both are good for the health of the vaginal wall muscles. The vaginal wall absorbs the ingredients present in the virgin olive oil and it aids in

healing atrophic vaginitis, dryness, loose vagina. Virgin Olive oil also has very low acidity. 1% or under 2% acidity is and may be safe. Extra virgin olive oil is readily available from pharmacies, drug stores and high-quality health food stores.

ALMOND OIL

Almond oil contains high levels of Vitamin E, is also a great source of estrogen. Almond oil can be applied on the vaginal walls to provide moisturizing effect. The vaginal walls will gradually absorb the component ingredients of the oil to restore moisture, and the health of the vaginal wall muscles, and with time restore the natural moisture supply by the vaginal muscles.

****

NOTE: *To this point, all the methods, techniques, foods and natural herbs, as discussed herein are to the best of our knowledge 99.9% safe without side and or after effect. Good thing about the information to this point is that you don't need to get old to start applying them. In fact, the earlier you start them and apply them throughout life the better. In all, maintaining a healthy and mindful lifestyle and incorporating the foods, herbs and exercise discussed thus far in your daily way of life should be a primary focus. The understanding that it is a continuous course of duty will make the intake of these vitamins and minerals to be effective in increasing and maintaining your vaginal health. The methods and techniques are not any quick fix. They take days, weeks, months and years to show a lasting effect.*

****

BF

CHAPTER 7.

VAGINA TIGHTENING CREAMS, GELS, SPEAYS

Vagina tightening creams, gels and sprays are made from ingredients that have skin tightening properties. Such ingredients include: Aloe, Oak gall, and some Vaseline, Olive Oil, Vitamin E. The creams, gels and sprays when applied regularly, and IF they contain real natural and active ingredients without components that will cause dryness and relapse if use is stopped, may be capable of helping the vagina regain its original shape and size/diameter. Most of the creams and gels have been advertised as helping to contract vaginal muscles and enhancing tightness and feeling of penetration for both partners. The creams, gels and sprays have been said to be free from side effects and after effects. Vagina tightening creams, gels and sprays are available in drug stores and pharmacies. Major source of ingredients used in Vagina tightening creams, gels and sprays include:

- ❖ Oak Gall
- ❖ Peuraria Mirifica
- ❖ Aloe

- ❖ Witch Hazel
- ❖ Vaseline
- ❖ Olive Oil
- ❖ Vitamin E

They may also contain other ingredients and petrochemical extracts such as:

- ➢ Glycerin
- ➢ Carbopol
- ➢ Propylene
- ➢ Butylene glycol

Some tightening creams, gels and spray may contain Alum and other obnoxious ingredients that may offer instant and temporary tightening or feeling of tightness by drawing out moisture from the walls of the vagina. However, they will later cause other problems such as Ph imbalance, vaginal bacterial floral death, and dryness. For best result, employ all methods laid out in this guide for tightening your loose and dry vagina including:

- ➢ Most especially do your Kegels with or without using the devices
- ➢ Use the natural oils for lubrication
- ➢ Consume foods and fruits with phytoestrogens
- ➢ Use the creams and gels when need be

Having a tight vagina is nothing difficult, you just have to want to have it so badly and you have to follow the guide religiously. And you can sexually enslave your man, enrich your sex life, improve and enhance your orgasm.

BF

CHAPTER 8

ALUM MISCONCEPTION – ALUM MYTH

During research and interview stage of writing this guide, we interviewed tens of people who attested that Alum worked for them in tightening their vagina. However, it is good to note that having your vagina temporarily tight and or getting your partner to have a little difficulty in travelling down the vaginal canal is not the same as having a tight, toned and healthy vaginal muscles. Sex workers also confessed to using it daily to tighten their vagina, however, all of them also said that they need vaginal lubricants to be able to effect safe/smooth penetration and lubricated intercourse. Remember, as we discussed in the earlier chapters, when the vaginal wall muscles are healthy, they are also toned. They are strong and ooze moisture into the vaginal canal. The ability to self-lubricate the vaginal canal is a sign of healthy vaginal wall muscles. All the sex workers and all the women interviewed also confessed that although there was general feeling of tightness of the vagina, they were not able to:

> ➤ Use the vaginal wall muscle and love muscles to clamp, clench,

massage and release the penis of their customers or loved ones at will

➢ Attain orgasm at all
➢ Attain orgasm any sooner
➢ Have orgasm more intense than usual
➢ Control their orgasm and that of their sex partner
➢ Control the session

Alum is a chemical compound called hydrated potassium aluminum sulphate. Alum has strong antiseptic properties. Alum has never been known to consist of nutrient(s) that nourish, tone, strengthen, aid circulation of blood, lubricate, and or rejuvenates the epithelial cells and or tissues of the skin, flesh or muscle. The vaginal wall muscles and the PC muscles though are finer, and invisible, but are not any different from the visible muscles of the biceps, calf, thigh, stomach and or shoulder muscles. The said muscles could not be toned, strengthened and or tightened by topically rubbing a chemical substance on them. Rather they could be toned, strengthened and tightened through training like you have in the gym, supplying them with nutrients that nourish and make them grow and respond to training and exercise. You must hold your vaginal wall muscles and PC muscles to the same standard. Employ Kegel exercise, foods, herbs, phytoestrogens, hormones, vitamins and grade oils.

It is very true that Alum is widely used to coagulate blood, like in after shaving, also used in vaccines to enhance the body's response to antigens, and can in some cases cause some temporary contraction. The very properties that aid Alum in its stop-bleeding (coagulation) ability could also make it to negate the moisture-oozing ability of the vaginal walls leading to dryness of the vaginal canal and may in prolonged usage and application lead to atrophic vaginitis which is a proud symptom of loose vagina.

However, it is also true that the strong antiseptic properties of Alum could be irritating, numbing and could upset the Ph balance of the vaginal canal. The strong anti-septic properties of Alum could bring about the extermination of the microbial flora or colony of the vaginal canal which is an integral part of vaginal health. The attendant ph imbalance may cause growth of bacterial pathogens in the vaginal canal, including yeast infections which will lead to vaginal odor, itching, vaginal dryness (which is a symptom of loose vagina as discussed in the early chapters). Therefore, for your health and safety, Alum should not and must not be used in the female genital.

****

PART 4

VAGINAL REJUVINATION

RECONSTRUCTIVE SURGERY

MEDICAL PROCEDURES

BF

CHAPTER 9

VAGINAL REJUVINATION

Throughout the pages of this book to this point, we pointed out ways that will aid you to maintain a tight healthy vagina. However, some women like a quick and immediate fix to their vaginal problems. Vaginal reconstructive surgery is not bad in itself, but the vagina is a very sensitive part of the woman's body and any surgery must be as a last resort and or very carefully considered, and if possible only when necessary. In being a sensitive part of the woman's body, the vagina undoubtedly has several nerves, nerve endings, receptors in the vaginal area that contribute to sexual health, sex drive, sexual well-being and orgasm. The possibility of any of the numerous nerves being mistakenly cut into, numbed and maybe cause permanent loss of sensation, and feel in the clitoris and vagina looms at every vaginal reconstructive surgery. This may result in a greater lack of sexual pleasure. According to experts interviewed during the course of writing this book, it is believed that those who are overweight, smoke cigarettes or suffer from Diabetes stand a greater risk of suffering complications resulting from reconstructive vaginal surgery.

Sometimes vaginal reconstructive surgery is performed for health reason while in other cases it is performed for cosmetic purposes. What should be expected after vaginal reconstructive surgery includes swelling and pain and discomfort may last up to three weeks. In general, most surgical procedure has its risks, but, healthcare experts state that vaginoplasty has a low rate of complications.

Most vaginal reconstructive surgery is performed under conscious sedation with local anesthetic, or general anesthetic. It is normally performed under 2hours, within a day.

VAGINAL REJUVENATION SURGERY

In vaginal rejuvenation surgeries, the procedure is used to re-tone and restructure flabby vaginal muscle. This may be achieved by removing some internal vaginal lining, 'excess' tissue, muscle tightening and repairing the vaginal muscles and wall, to restore the muscle tone and tightness of the vagina.

However, some women complained about scarring, infection and also a loss of sexual sensation around the clitoris. Other side effect or complications of Vaginaplasty include Anorgasmia – difficulty to achieve orgasm, Sexual desire disorder. For More Info about Anorgasmia and sexual desire disorder see the Book **Bedroom Logic** By Be Your Dream Press.

Some Side Effects of Reconstructive Surgery

- ❖ Anorgasmia
- ❖ Loss of pleasure or sensation
- ❖ Scarring
- ❖ numbness

❖ Pain upon intercourse

❖ Hematoma

❖ Infection

LABIAPLASTY: This is the surgical reconstruction of the vaginal labia. This procedure is mainly performed for cosmetic purposes. Labial surgery can be used to reduce the labia of some women who have naturally large or whose labia disproportionally enlarged after two or more childbirths.

The labia minor are the flaps of skin directly either side of the vagina. Large labia minor may be a source of irritation and even stop some women from wearing tight dresses and tight pants.

HOODECTOMY

This is mostly done for esthetics purposes. This surgical procedure reduces or removes the hood of the clitoris. It's been said that this surgical procedure helps to improve sexual sensation/sensitivity around the clitoris.

LIPOSUCTION

This procedure is used to remove excess fat from the woman's vulva. In other cases, a fuller and fatter vulva may be what is desired in a liposuction, in which case fat grafting can be performed.

****

CAUTION!

Before deciding to have a vaginal reconstructive surgery, put in a great deal of thought into it to make sure it is worth it and that you cannot achieve it by the other methods outlined in the pages of this book. You also need to put just as much thought into selecting a clinic where the reconstructive surgery has to be performed and the qualification/certification of the surgeon to perform the procedure? Remember, you are about to undertake a potentially life-changing procedure, and you surely want to employ the best professional services and facilities available.

Check with your Country's:

Association of Plastic and Reconstructive Surgeons

Cosmetic Surgeons Association

Cosmetic Plastic Surgeons Association

Or whatever the association or council is known with.

You may also check with the International Society of Aesthetic Plastic Surgery. These bodies will be glad to offer your information about their member surgeons and clinics.

****

GENERAL BRIEF

In the general politics of any relationship, and marriage, the politics of the bedroom is the most vital. Guess Why? Because once you and your sex partner are happy each time you embark on your journey to heaven, to paradise, the rest of the drag that is present in any relationship becomes manageable.

However, it is very good that you understand that the bedroom fool is the real fool of any relationship, notwithstanding educational level, wealth and intelligence. All the points, methods, techniques, foods, vitamins and minerals outlined in this book are not quick fix. Maintaining a healthy and mindful lifestyle and incorporating the foods, herbs and exercise discussed in this edition of the book, in your daily way of life should be a primary focus. The understanding that it is a continuous course of duty and lifestyle will make the intake of these food, herbs, vitamins and minerals to be effective in increasing and maintaining your vaginal health. For best result, articulate feeding with doing your Kegel exercise. Some of the herbs are better used on intermittent rather than on a daily basis. Again, as said earlier, the methods and techniques are not any quick fix. They take days, weeks, months and years to show a lasting effect. Good thing about the manifestation of the result/effect of the exercise and dietary regimen is that once they manifest, most people can hold on for as long as life permits. Why? Because you will get used to doing your Kegels, and maintaining a dietary regimen.

GLOSSARY OF TERMS

Vaginal muscles – the muscles (flesh) lining the vaginal canal

Stratified – having layers, not a solid whole

Epithelial – membranous tissues of one or more layers of cells, always having protective or covering functions.

Anterior wall – front wall

Posterior wall – back wall

Vaginal canal – the hole inside the vagina

Elastin – structural protein responsible for the elasticity of the vagina, penis and skin

Vaginal muscularis – vaginal smooth muscles

PC muscle – Pelvic muscle (aka Love muscle)

Estrogen – female sex hormone (also present in men in smaller quantity)

Incontinence - inability to stop urine leakage from the bladder, the loss of control over the muscle that controls the bladder (aperture) opening and closure

Menopause – the phase when a woman stops seeing her menstrual cycle, stop ovulating.

Vaginal atrophy – the thinning and wasting away of the vaginal wall/vaginal muscle

Structural changes – changes in the structure, shape, form

Bladder – the human urine sac

Bladder muscle – the muscle that controls the opening and closing of the bladder for the passage of urine

Rectal wall muscles – the muscles lining the rectal canal

Rectum – the tube through which stool is pushed out to the outside as you defecate

Vaginal Prolapse – vaginal collapse, when all the muscles became loose, and the bladder or rectum falls into the vaginal canal

Flatulence – outing of air

Vaginal Flatulence – expelling air from the vagina (vaginal farting)

Kegels – name given to vaginal wall muscle exercise as an attribute to Dr. Kegel who developed/discovered the exercise in the 1940's

Kegel Exercise - name given to vaginal wall muscle and PC muscle exercise as an attribute to Dr. Kegel who developed/discovered the exercise in the 1940's

Kegel balls – Devices and objects developed over the years to help target the exact PC muscle as you perform Kegels

Pelvic Floor - The pelvic floor is that point in the pelvic region of the body where all the connective tissues and muscles that support all the organs of the pelvis connects

Hormones – Bio-chemicals (chemicals of the body) in the body system that affects body changes and functions

Hormonal changes – changes in the levels of the body hormones

Testosterone – the male sex hormone, it helps give the male characteristics

Stinging Wasp – an insect

Symptom – manifested sign

Phytoestrogen – estrogens that are naturally present in plants

Estrogen-like chemicals – chemicals that resemble estrogen

Estrogenic activities – activities native to estrogens

Neurotransmitters – Body electrical transmitters

Omega-3 fatty acids – they are not acids in the common sense of the word acid. It is the name given to some essential fats that is good for the body system

Optimum hormonal level – perfect level for the body estrogen, a level at which it is at its best

Hormonal imbalance – imbalance of the levels of the hormones in the body system

Progesterone – a sex hormone present in both male and female body system, always more in males than females

Testosterone - a sex hormone present in both males and females, often more in men. Testosterone is responsible for sex drive/libido. It is sometimes called libido hormone

Muscular contraction and relaxation – the ease and squeeze actions/movements of the body muscles

Roe – Fish eggs harvested for food

***** ***** ***** *****

ABOUT BE-YOUR-DREAM PRESS

Be your dream press is an imprint of Obrake USA LLC. We are publishers of non-fiction books. Books published by Be Your Dream Press are mainly books that help people to be whatever they want to be, to become their dreams. Books that help people succeed in doing whatever legitimate thing they want to engage in. Be Your Dream Press publishes series of health and beauty books, women health books and the very popular series called Financial Democracy Series.

Books by **Be Your Dream Books** Include:

BEDROOM POLITICS SERIES

- ➤ Bedroom Justice
- ➤ Bedroom Logic
- ➤ Bedroom Wisdom

HEALTH and BEAUTY SERIES

- ➤ Secrets To Skin Glow and Radiance
- ➤ Secrets To Hair Growth and Sheen

FINANCIAL DEMOCRACY SERIES

- ❖ A Manufacturer Without A Factory
- ❖ Steps to Sell, Supply and Do Business with New York City
- ❖ Steps to Sell, Supply and Do Business with Large Corporations in America
- ❖ Steps to Sell, Supply and Do Business with Educational Institutions in America
- ❖ Steps to Sell, Supply and Do Business with International Institutions and Organizations

❖ Dozen Businesses You Can Start and Run in America

For more information visit us at: www.obrake.com

OTHER BOOKS BY BeYourDream Press

FINANCIAL DEMOCRACY SERIES – CANADA

➢ Two Dozen Businesses You Can Start and Run in Canada

➢ No Canadian Experience

FINANCIAL DEMOCRACY SERIES – SOUTH AFRICA

❖ Steps to Sell, Supply and Do Business with National, Provincial, Local and Municipal Government of South Africa

❖ Steps to Sell, Supply and Do Business with Public and Private Corporations in South Africa

❖ How to Start and Run Your Business in South Africa

❖ Two Dozen Businesses You Can Start and Run in South Africa

❖ When South African Banks Say No

Visit us at: www.obrake.com

Bedroom Politics Series

THE BEDROOM FOOL

The Bedroom Fool is the Real Fool of Any Relationship!

In general, the politics of a relationship is a complex one.

However, one aspect of the general politics of any relationship is outstanding and it is the **Bedroom Politics**.

In this arena of politics, do not let your guard down; if you fail in this section, you lose everything. **Don't Be The Bedroom Fool!** Oftentimes, women for different reasons want to tighten and rejuvenate their vagina. No matter the reason, truth is tightening your vaginal and pc muscles will enhance your sex life, improve your self-esteem and may help relationship with your partner. **No Matter How Beautiful, Educated or Rich You May Be**, If You are a Bedroom Fool, you will find it hard to keep partners for the long sweet haul and or keep them faithful to you, sexually. Sexual faithfulness for the most part is by virtue of sexual satisfaction with a partner. **The Secret to tightening, elasticizing and rejuvenating your vaginal and pc muscles is well laid out in this guide. In this edition you will find how to:**

> - Be Able to Clamp and Clench with Vaginal Muscles
> - Be Able to Squeeze-Massage-Ease-Release
> - Tighten Your Vaginal Muscle
> - Learn Vagina Muscle Exercise
> - Restore Your Vaginal Teenage Elasticity
> - Reverse Your Genital Aging Clock
> - Be Healthy and Beautiful Between Your Legs
> - Improve Sex Life Multifold by Strengthening Vaginal Muscles
> - Become Truly Irresistible To Your Partner

Visit us at: www.obrake.com

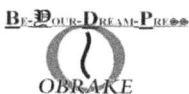

Be-Your-Dream-Press

OBRAKE

www.ingramcontent.com/pod-product-compliance
Lightning Source LLC
Chambersburg PA
CBHW020006290326
41935CB00007B/321